NUTRITION AND HEALTH
The Vegetarian Way

Of Allied Interest

1. Speaking of: Nature Cure
   K. L. Sarma & S. Swaminathan
2. Speaking of Yoga — A Practical Guide
   Pt. Shambunath
3. Speaking of Yoga and Nature Cure Therapy
   K. S. Joshi
4. Yoga: An Easy Approach
   Prem Bhatia
5. Stress Management through Yoga and Meditation
   Pt. Shambunath
6. योग एक सहज प्रयास
   प्रेम भाटिया

All you wanted to know about

1. Yoga for Health and Happiness
   Dr. Savitri Ramaiah   Rs. 50
2. Sun Therapy
   Vijaya Kumar   Rs. 50
3. Yoga
   Lalitha Sharma   Rs. 50
4. Healing Powers of Water
   Dr. Savitri Ramaiah   Rs. 50
5. Acupressure in Daily Life
   Dr. Savitri Ramaiah   Rs. 50
6. Nutrition
   Dr. Savitri Ramaiah   Rs. 50

Published by
Sterling Publishers Private Limited

NUTRITION AND HEALTH
The Vegetarian Way

 **Institute of Naturopathy
& Yogic Sciences, Bangalore   A Sterling Paperback**

STERLING PAPERBACKS
An imprint of
Sterling Publishers (P) Ltd.
A-59, Okhla Industrial Area, Phase-II,
New Delhi-110020.
Tel: 26387070, 26386209; Fax: 91-11-26383788
E-mail: sterlingpublishers@airtelbroadband.in
ghai@nde.vsnl.net.in
www.sterlingpublishers.com

INSTITUTE OF NATUROPATHY & YOGIC SCIENCES
Jindal Nagar, Tumkur Road, Bangalore 560073
Ph: 8394926, 8396337 Fax No 91 80-8396339
Email: inys@satyam.net.in
Website: http://www.naturecure-inys.org

NUTRITION AND HEALTH: The Vegetarian Way
© 2002, Institute of Naturopathy & Yogic Sciences, Bangalore
ISBN 81 207 2424 0
Reprint 2005, 2006, 2007

All rights are reserved.
No part of this publication may be reproduced, stored in a retrieval
system or transmitted, in any form or by any means, mechanical,
photocopying, recording or otherwise, without prior written
permission of the original publisher.

Printed and Published by Sterling Publishers Pvt. Ltd., New Delhi-110 020.

Foreword

Life cannot be sustained without food, which is, in fact, one of the basic needs of life, the other two being air and water. Man needs sufficient nourishment for growth, development and maintenance of health.

What we eat matters greatly for the maintenance of normal health and prevention of diseases. Many diseases of the modern day, such as obesity, diabetes, coronary heart diseases, low backaches, high BP, asthma, arthritis and migraine are all the result of digestive disorders, and have their roots in the kind of food we eat, and the way it is prepared or processed.

Advancement of science and technology in preserving, canning, processing and producing foods has certainly added varieties of convenient foods, but certain methods have proved to be fatal to the human body and the safety of a few others is still suspected.

Chemical fertilizers sprayed with alarming casualness in farming, gases used for artificial ripening of fruits, and preservatives used for canning, results in our consuming quite a lot of chemicals, prolonged intake of which is definitely harmful. There is, therefore, need to cultivate the habit of eating fresh foods, as far as possible. Proper nutrition and adoption of sensible eating habits can surely reduce the risk of illness.

Fruits and vegetables in their natural form are the best diet of man, for which he is physiologically most fit. Man can develop great resistance to disease with this diet and a regular healthy lifestyle. Utmost care is to be taken while cooking. It should be borne in mind that for the sake of taste, we should not deviate from the basic purpose of food, which is nourishment.

With the above in mind, the Institute of Naturopathy and Yogic Sciences has brought out this book to give you an idea as to what is to be eaten and when and how. Please do not forget Palm C.Bragg's dictum: "You are what you eat."

K. R. Raghunath
Chairman (INYS)

Preface

A very natural sequel to the unique experience of all the patients at this Institute is the question - "Doctor, what should I eat, and what should I avoid eating when I get back home?"

This book makes an attempt to answer such queries. It is designed to serve as a guide not only for the sick, but also for the convalescent and the healthy. The last chapter deals with recipes ideal for patients.

The dishes suggested are flavoury, tasty, nourishing and appealing with their natural colours.

Patients who have undergone nature cure treatments and advised to continue a follow-up diet should avoid excessively spicy ingredients in the preparations. Most of the preparations will be tasty even with very less spices.

These preparations are suggested bearing in mind the fundamental and potent role the diet plays in promoting health and happiness.

In this connection, it is necessary to bear the following in mind:

1. Fruits are naturally cooked by sun's rays when they ripen and hence easily digestible. They help cleanse the body too.
2. Sprouts, raw vegetable, salads and fruits are living foods, more beneficial than cooked foods.
3. It is vital to adopt the correct cooking techniques to minimize the loss of nutrients, which occurs during traditional and unscientific cooking methods.
4. Eat only when you are hungry.
5. Overeating causes indigestion and leads to diseases.
6. Drink your solid food and eat your liquid food.

It is time we adopt 'Eat to live' attitude rather than 'Live to eat'.

Wishing you a more nutritious life.

Naturally yours,
Dr. S. N. Murthy
Chief Medical Officer

CONTENTS

PART I
GENERAL NUTRITION

PART II
THERAPEUTIC NUTRITION

PART III
RECIPES

PART 1

GENERAL NUTRITION

1

Foods and Nutrients

Good health largely depends on the nutrition. To sustain life and perform various functions, man needs a wide range of nutrients, including proteins, fats, carbohydrates, vitamins and minerals. These are the chemical substances derived from the food. The food we eat daily, classified as cereals, pulses, legumes, nuts, oil seeds, vegetables, fruits, milk and milk products, consist of all the nutrients.

Food in general is grouped into two nutritive, which provides energy, heat and nutrition and non-nutritive, providing only energy.

Vitamins and minerals: Vitamins and minerals do not supply energy, but play a very important role in the regulation of metabolic activities. Minerals are useful in the formation of body structure and skeleton.

Carbohydrates: Carbohydrates provide energy to the body and help control breakdown of proteins and protect it from toxins. Even to burn the fat, the presence of carbohydrate is very essential.

Glucose which is otherwise known as monosaccharide, is the basic chemical that provides energy to the body. These are simple sugars which get easily converted into energy, for example: sugar, honey, jaggery etc.

Polysaccharides are made of many single glucose molecules, of which starch is the most important. It is commonly referred to as complex carbohydrate. When a diet rich in complex carbohydrates is consumed, glucose molecules present in them break up to supply the energy requirement. Complex carbohydrates are generally found in cereals, grains, vegetables and fruits. Since complex carbohydrates take a longer time to digest than the simple ones, they are more effective in controlling hunger.

Proteins: Proteins are called building stones. Proteins are various combinations of essential amino acids. They are grouped as simple, compound and derived proteins.

Simple proteins are substances which when dissolved in water breakdown into amino acids. *Compound proteins* are a combination of simple proteins, with some other non-protein substances. *Derived proteins* are formed at various stages of the breakdown of simple and compound proteins.

To maintain life and promote growth, proteins which are complete, are very essential. Complete proteins keep one alive, but do not support growth.

The dietary proteins are broken down into amino acids and absorbed as such, and the body synthesises them again into proteins, as and when required.

All foods, except refined sugar, oil and fats contain proteins in varying degrees. Milk, oilseeds, nuts and pulses contain a good amount of protein. Soyabean is a rich source of protein.

Proteins are required for maintaining the wear and tear of the tissues in adults, for growth in infants and children, for foetal development during pregnancy and milk generation during lactation. An adult requires protein to the extent of O.7 gm/kg of the body weight, if the protein quality is good, while requirement should be 1 gm/kg of body weight if one takes a mixed vegetable diet. Children during growing age require slightly more proteins than adults.

Fats: Fat is an essential part of the diet, but taken in excess, is harmful to the body. Fat generally breaks up in the absence of carbohydrates to provide energy. Since fat is a concentrated source of energy, any excess intake of fat can lead to fat accumulation, which is termed as "obesity".

The fat that we eat consists of fatty acids. Fat is very important for absorbing vitamins like A,D,E and K. The body needs fat for growth and repair. The fat accumulated in the tissues gives shape and cushioning effect to the body and acts as an insulator. Fat also helps in regulating body temperature.

The most important aspect of dietary fat is its degree of the saturation. The higher the saturation, the greater the chances of accumulation of cholesterol in the body, which leads to heart diseases. Hence, fat which contains more polyunsaturated fatty acids is preferred to the one that contains saturated fatty acids. Good sources of polyunsaturated fatty acids are: safflower oil, sunflower oil, corn oil, soyabean oil, olive oil etc.

Generally, Indians consume regularly about 40-50 per cent of calories as fat. Contrary to the popular belief, taking starch does not cause obesity. Eating too much fat makes one obese because each gram of fat yields twice the amount of energy, generally produced by carbohydrates and proteins.

Cholesterol: Cholesterol is a waxy substance which forms the essential part of the body cell walls. It also helps in the production of vitamins, hormones, bile acids and nerve tissues. It moves in the blood stream after its synthesis in the form of lipoproteins. Most of the cholesterol is synthesised in the body itself and only 15 per cent of it is derived from the diet. That is the reason why even after a severe diet restriction, only a very low reduction in the total cholesterol levels is seen.

The body continues to synthesise cholesterol regardless of the intake of diet. Hence, excess cholesterol is deposited in the blood vessels narrowing them and causing heart disease.

The type of lipoprotein by which cholesterol is transported is also an important factor for heart disease. The cholesterol in the blood is of 3 types, low density lipoprotein (LDL), which is present in the blood stream and contributes to cholesterol levels, the very low density lipoprotein (VLDL),which carries cholesterol from cell to cell and the high density lipoprotein (HDL), which generally takes cholesterol to intestines for final disposal from the body. Hence, the higher the HDL cholesterol, the higher the protection from heart attacks. In contrast, the higher the LDL cholesterol, the greater is the risk of heart diseases.

The ideal method to maintain total cholesterol level is to increase the HDL cholesterol by increasing the intake of high fibre food. Regular exercise also lowers the LDL cholesterol levels. Another way of maintaining cholesterol level is to cut down intake of fat to the minimum, particularly saturated fats. Non-vegetarian food is to be restricted.

Fibre: There are two kinds of fibre, soluble and insoluble. Fibre is the non-digestible part of the plant food which consists of mainly complex carbohydrates. Fibre is generally found in whole grains, legumes, fruits and vegetables. Fibre is removed when the food is refined and processed. Non-vegetarian food contains no fibre.

Soluble fibre:

Soluble fibre forms gels that delay the absorption of certain foods, including cholesterol, sugar etc. It is found in oat bran, rice bran, rolled oats, carrots and pectins (found in fruit), psyllium and gourgum (found in beans), and mucillagenous fibre present in fenugreek (methi). Soluble fibre increases excretion of cholesterol and also regulates blood glucose levels by delaying absorption of carbohydrates.

Insoluble fibre:

This increases the bulk of stool and substantially reduces the time taken for food to pass through intestines. The increase in bulk relieves constipation, as food travels faster through the intestines and is less exposed to toxins. Wheat bran is a major source of insoluble fibre.

2

The Digestion of Food

If the food we eat is to be assimilated by the body, it must undergo a number of physical and chemical changes in the digestive system. The main function of the digestive system is to break down carbohydrates, proteins and fats into simpler substances for proper absorption of the same, to keep the body systems working, and also expel the residual waste as faeces.

The process of digestion includes mechanical and chemical processes. Mechanical process of digestion includes:

- Chewing of food
- Swallowing of food
- Churning of food
- Contraction of the intestinal tract

Chemical process involves mixing up of water with the food, and splitting it later on. The chemical process is speeded up by the enzymes, which are secreted in the mouth (i.e. salivary juice), in the stomach (gastric juice), and in the small intestine (combination of bile acids and bile juice secreted by the liver, pancreatic juice and intestinal juice).

Digestion in the mouth: Food is broken down by chewing and swallowed after it is moistened with the saliva. Digestion begins at this stage. Most of the digestion of carbohydrates is completed in the mouth itself.

Digestion in the stomach: The mixed food is passed on to the stomach via the oesophagus or the food pipe. The stomach temporarily acts as a store house for food. The hydrochloric acid present in the stomach acts as a protective barrier against micro-organisms present in the food, swells protein for its easy digestion, and provides acid media necessary for the action of pepsin.

Pepsin, a protein splitting enzyme present in the gastric juice, partially digests protein. It also digests milk through the enzyme, renin. Very little conversion of carbohydrates and fats take place in the stomach.

The semi-digested, properly mixed food in the form of semi-solid mass chyme is passed on to the small intestines for further conversion.

Digestion in the small intestine: As soon as the food is passed on to the first part of the small intestine (the duodenum), bile juice from the gall bladder and at the same time, pancreatic juice from the pancreas are released and both juices flow into the duodenum. Bile emulsifies fat which is later on digested properly and neutralises the acidity by providing alkalinity. The pancreatic juice acts on partially digested protein to convert it into amino acids, partially digested carbohydrates into simple sugars, and emulsified fat into fatty acids and glycerols.

Here in the duodenum complete digestion of food takes place and the rest is passed on to the last part of the intestine, the ileum, where useful contents of the food are absorbed and the rest are passed on into the large intestine where the refuse mixes with water in the 10-foot-long colon for the final evacuation as faeces, through the rectum and anus.

Acidity of food

There are several kinds of acids present in the food, of which three found in natural foods are utilised by the body. These three acids are citric, malic and tartaric acids. The other acids formed are harmful and are not utilised by the body. They are oxalic, benzoic, butyric and uric acids. There is another acid called lactic acid, which is not utilised by the body but is protective in nature. *Citric acid* is present in lemons, oranges, grapefruit, gooseberries and pomegranate fruits, and in tomato, radish and other vegetables. Malic acid is found in apples, peas, grapes and tomatoes. Tartaric acid is found in grapes and in small amounts in pineapple.

Acetic acid is present in vinegar and in soya sauce, and is harmful during digestion. Oxalic acid found in spinach, rhuburb, cocoa, tea and pepper is harmful, more so, if one has the tendency to higher uric acid levels leading to gout.

Benzoic acid is present in prunes, plums and berries. People with a tendency to uric acid, calculi of bladder or kidney should avoid foods containing these acids. Benzoic acid is also used as a preservative in canned fruits, apple cider. vinegar and sauces.

Butyric acid is present in butter and fat, turned rancid. It is highly irritating to the stomach and often gives rise to acidosis.

Uric acid is one of the waste products of the body. Non-vegetarian food sources produce large quantities of uric acid. Spinach, beans, peas, cauliflower and mushrooms also contain purines which later produce uric acid, moderately. People with gout arthritis and having tendency to urinary stone formation should use these vegetables moderately.

Alkalinity of food

Oxidation of food within the body results in the formation of a residue or ash. Most of the time people with acidity avoid citrus fruits, out of fear that it might lead to acidity. On the contrary, fresh fruits contain organic acids, which are readily utilised by the body leaving alkaline traces. Anything natural, the system receives well.

By taking milk, fruits, vegetables in plenty and reducing on cereals, non-vegetarian sources, pulses, legumes, etc., one can keep up alkalinity for maintaining good health of the internal system.

In other words, by eating a well balanced diet, one can strike a balance between acidity and alkalinity in the internal system, which is essential for health. The cardinal rule for maintaining acid-alkali balance is eating 40 per cent cereals and 60 per cent fruits and vegetables in the daily diet.

3

The Calorie Theory - Energy from Food

The food we eat yields energy which is measured by a unit called 'calorie'.

Although we eat varieties of food prepared in different ways, it is finally the energy produced by it for the utilisation of the body cells that counts. Different kinds of food produce different quantum of energy depending on the energy giving substances they contain, such as carbohydrates, fats and protein. Each gram of carbohydrate and protein produces 4 calories of energy and 9 calories of fat whereas 1 gm of alcohol produces roughly 7 calories. Water, dietary fibre, vitamins, minerals and condiments produce no calories. Sugar and sweets provide only energy and no nutrition. Hence they are called 'empty calories. Some of the food high in fat content such as butter, alcohol, chocolate, hydrogenated oils, fried foods etc. are high calorific substances.

The energy requirements of a person for 24 hours can be standardised based on (i) the basal metabolism (ii) energy spent in exercises and work (iii) utilisation of food and, (iv) growth if any.

Based on these, the daily energy requirement of an average sedentary male of 55 kg. weight is put at 2400 kcal/day minimum, whereas that of a sedentary female of 45 kg. weight at 1900 kcal/day.

According to the calorie theory, the energy we need for daily activities is derived from the diet we eat. If this theory is true, then probably, when we do not eat, we will have no energy for our activities. That means when the patient is bedridden or ill he must be fed to keep his strength which, according to Naturopathy, is not acceptable. In fact, during acute illness, abstinence from food or fasting is judiciously employed to help the patient overcome illness. The body then derives its energy from the food stored in the body, which can be proved by the example that, when a person undertakes fast he survives till the stored food is exhausted. This shows clearly that the calorie theory is a confusing one.

From the rational dietetics point of view, it is considered that, a balanced diet comprising fresh, wholesome, unprocessed foods, and in particular raw foods can provide enough energy for survival, though in terms of actual calories it is offering less than actually needed.

Taking into consideration the age, sex, weight, height, body frame, body activity and temperature, mental activity, climatic changes etc., it is now quite evident, that no formula which is foolproof could be evolved for feeding the human body

Calorie is only a yardstick to measure the food quantity but it tells nothing about the quality. So, one should not only count the calories while eating, but should also look into the nutritive value of the food.

4

Food Groups

In order to remain healthy we have to obtain all the essential nutrients such as carbohydrates, proteins, fats, minerals, trace elements etc. from the diet. No single food item supplies all the necessary nutrients human body requires. Hence the need to eat different foods to meet the nutrients requirement cannot be overlooked.

I

The major food stuffs that make a typical Indian diet and their nutritional contributions are discussed below:

a) **Cereals and millets:** Major cereals and millets consumed in India are rice, wheat, jowar, bajra and ragi. The cereals are the major source of energy and on an average we derive 70-80 per cent of our energy from cereals and millets. Cereals contain 50-60 per cent carbohydrates and 6-12 per cent proteins. Cereals are also a good source of calcium and iron. Ragi especially is a very rich source of calcium. Cereals too are important sources of vitamin B. Since they are present in the outer brown layer of the cereal, refining or polishing removes the amount of vitamin B available from the cereal. Cereals are also rich in fibre.

b) **Pulses:** These are rich sources of protein in our diets. Particularly for vegetarians, pulses are very important, because they are the only important source of protein. Major pulses found in Indian diets include bengalgram, blackgram, greengram, cowpea, horsegram, kesaridal, lentil, mothpeas, rajma, redgram and soyabean. Some of them are used as dals as well as whole grains.

c) **Fruits and vegetables:**

Fruits: They deserve an important place in our daily diet, since these are easily digestible and easily acceptable to the system in their natural form. Fruits are very important because of their alkaline properties, high percentage of moisture content and low fat and protein content.

Fruits are mainly divided into sweet sub-acid and acid fruits. The nutrients present in the fruits can best be obtained by the body, if fruits are thoroughly masticated.

Fruits are generally good sources of vitamins. Indian gooseberry (amla) and guava are rich sources of vitamin C. Yellow-coloured fruits like mango and papaya contain carotene (pro-vitamin A). Banana and mosambi (sweet lime) are rich in potassium. Fruits also contain pectin which provides bulk to the diet and helps in easier bowel evacuation.

Dried fruits such as figs, dates, raisins are good sources of iron. A very good way to eat fruits is to take it as a meal in itself. One should not eat fruit along with the normal meal.

Vegetables: Many types of green leafy vegetables are consumed daily in our country. The one commonly used are: palak, amaranth, fenugreek (*methi*), drumstick (*saijan patta*), mint (*pudina*), mustard, dil etc. The green leafy vegetables are excellent sources of calcium, iron and carotene (pro-vitamin A), vitamin C, vitamin B2 and folic acid. Green leafy vegetables are inexpensive and very useful for growth and maintenance of general health. These must be consumed by children and pregnant women as additional supplements of nutrition required by them. Another advantage of these green leafy vegetables is that they are available throughout the year and are also easily grown in the kitchen gardens.

Roots and tubers: Some of the important root vegetables used in India are: potato, carrot, beetroot, sweet potato, yam, colocassia, tapioca, etc. They are all rich in carbohydrates (starch) and are important sources of energy. Carrots are rich in carotene and potato in vitamin C. Tapioca and yam are rich in calcium.

Other vegetables such as brinjal, all gourd varieties, beans, lady's finger, tomato etc. are very low in calories and supply a good amount of vitamins and minerals. Apart from this, vegetables are easily digestible and a good source of dietary fibre, providing bulk to the diet, which helps in easy evacuation.

d) **Nuts and oil seeds:** Like pulses, they are also rich in protein and contain high level of fat. Some of the commonly used nuts and oilseeds are; almond, cashewnut, pistachio, walnut etc. oilseeds, such as safflower, sunflower, gingerly, groundnut, coconut, mustard seed are used for extracting oils.

e) **Fats and oils:** Visible fats commonly consumed are butter, ghee, hydrogenated oils (Vanaspati) and various vegetable oils such as groundnut, safflower, sunflower, gingerly, mustard, coconut, soyabean, corn etc. All fats are concentrated sources of energy providing 9 kcal/g. Total calories from visible fat should not exceed 20 per cent of the intake of calories. Some of the vegetable oils high in polyunsaturated fatty acids should be preferred in the following order.

1. Safflower oil
2. Sunflower oil
3. Soyabean oil
4. Corn oil
5. Olive oil
6. Gingerly oil
7. Mustard oil
8. Groundnut oil
9. Coconut oil

f) **Milk and milk products:** This group covers milk, condensed milk, milk powder, paneer, cheese, cream, butter and fermented products like curds, buttermilk etc.

Milk is an ideal food for infants and children because it is a good source of protein, calcium and vitamin B2. However, milk is deficient in iron and vitamin C. Milk is suitable for infants and children during the growing age because an enzyme is produced during that period, which helps in assimilating the milk and as the growth stops, the enzyme production diminishes. Hence milk is not therapeutically prescribed in the case of adults.

When fat content of milk is removed, it is called skimmed milk and it is especially used by weight watchers and if moisture is removed from milk it becomes condensed milk, which is used in making sweets. Totally dried, powdered milk is used when fresh milk is not readily available.

Milk products such as cream, butter, cheese, paneer etc. also find a place in the Indian diet.

Fermented milk products such as curds and buttermilk are more easily digestible than sweet milk because of the lactic acid present in them. Curds and buttermilk are good for developing a healthy intestinal flora, hence they are used in treating all abdominal disorders.

g) **Condiments and spices:** These are accessory food substances used in minimal quantities in Indian diets as flavouring agents to improve palatability of food. Some of them are: green chillies, dry chillies, turmeric powder, mustard, onion, pepper, ginger, garlic, coriander, thyme, fennel seeds, cumin etc. Some of the spices such as turmeric, asafoetida, garlic have antibacterial property and inhibit growth of bacteria.

II

Salt

Salt is a major health hazard which affects our general health to the extent that it causes high blood pressure and coronary heart disease. An adult, as per the nutrition experts, needs only 1 gm of salt a day, but most of us consume far more than what is required. All fruits, vegetables, milk, cereals, grain, pulses, nuts etc. do contain small amounts of sodium. We get enough of it from these sources. Consumption of extra salt is not only unnecessary, but also hazardous to health. Some people easily excrete excess sodium through the kidneys and therefore it does not cause any harm to them. But for some people, who cannot excrete sodium in urine, raises their blood pressure. Such people are otherwise called salt sensitive individuals and they have to restrict salt. But reducing salt from diet benefits all, at least to some extent.

Another problem is, about three quarters of salt we eat goes through processed food. Flavour enhances like mono-sodium glutamate, baking powder (sodium bicarbonate), sodium cyclamate, sodium sacharin (artificial sweetner), sodium nitrate, sodium benzonate (preservative) do contain small quantities of sodium.

Tips to cut down salt:

- Do not add extra salt to cooked food and gradually reduce even that till your taste gets adjusted, and then maintain at minimum level.
- Use substitutes for salt such as lime juice, spices or herbs for flavour.
- Avoid highly salted foods such as potato chips, sauces, crisps, processed cheese, salted nuts, pickles, ketch-ups and soya sauces.
- Start salt restriction early in life. Better way is to develop the habit in childhood itself.

Sugar

Eating refined sugar raises blood sugar level rapidly. Despite the widespread knowledge that sugar causes dental caries and contributes to obesity, sugar consumption is still on the higher side throughout the world. Sugar is consumed directly and also in the form of cake, pastries, puddings, desserts, ice creams, sweets, carbonated drinks, fruit squashes, jams, marmalades etc.

Tips to cut down sugar:

- Drink unsweetened fresh fruit juices
- Do not eat sweets or restrict them to eating once in a while
- Eat fruits in between meals and not along with it.
- Eat a fruit as a snack instead of biscuits, chocolates etc.
- Reduce sugar in the recipes
- Avoid processed, sweetened foods.

Honey

Honey has very rightly been called the 'Food of Gods'. As one of the most ancient elixirs known to man, honey is universal in its appeal. It is popular for its medicinal properties too.

Honey being much more than a sweetener has been given a much higher position.

Composition of honey

Honey chiefly consists of sugars and water. It contains:

Water	17%
Levulose (D-fructose)	39%
Dextrose (D-glucose)	34%
Sucrose	1%
Dextrin	0.5%
Proteins	2%
Wax	1%
Plant acids (malic, formic, citric etc.)	0.5%
Salts (calcium, iron, phosphates, magnesium, iodine)	1%
Undetermined residues (resins, gums, pigments, volatile oils, pollen grains)	40%

The sugars found in honey are glucose, fructose and sucrose. *Glucose* is the simplest of all sugars, and can be assimilated directly by the blood.

Fructose is commonly called grape sugar. It is also known as levulose. Its chemical composition is similar to that of glucose. But, it crystallises more readily than glucose. While glucose helps in restoring the oxygen level, fructose builds the tissues.

Sucrose is a combination of fructose and glucose.

A little dextrin is found in honey. Dextrin is a gummy substance that can be assimilated by the blood directly and therefore easily digestible.

The amount of proteins in honey is very less. There are at least six vitamins in honey. These include: thiamin (vitamin B1), ascorbic acid (vitamin C), riboflavin, pantothenic acid, pyridoxine and niacin.

The vitamin contents present in honey vary depending upon the nectar source. As vitamins are present in very small amounts, repeated filtration usually removes them. Also vitamins would be destroyed when honey is heated or processed.

Benefits of honey

As a tonic:

One of the greatest energy-giving drinks given to us by nature is honey. Eating a spoonful of honey gives a person energy in less than ten minutes. The glycogen which passes into the blood stream gives us the same amount of energy which we obtain after taking a regular meal. It is often used as an energy giver in emergency cases like fatigue and exhaustion. Honey with fresh greens, fresh fruits, nuts' and milk, makes an ideal diet for good health and youthfulness.

Honey can be taken with milk, cream or butter. It is a restorative tonic after serious illness. Regular intake of honey goes a long way in maintaining good health.

If we compare the composition of honey and refined sugar, it is observed that honey contains more than two dozen vitamins and minerals, while refined sugar has none. Though refined sugar contains more calories than honey, it is harmful. Refined sugar is ultimately dangerous to the body.

Honey however, contains mainly levulose and glucose. While the glucose present is rapidly absorbed by the blood, levulose is assimilated slowly. This slower assimilation is, however, advantageous to the body as it does not lead to a sudden increase in the blood sugar level.

Honey unlike white sugar does not ferment in the digestive tract. Fermentation sets up ideal conditions for the growth of harmful bacteria . Partially digested, high starch content food also promotes growth of harmful bacteria.

Honey can also be used to treat boils and external sores.

Mixed with soap and applied on the boil, the mixture rapidly draws out the pus and the moisture present and thereby cleanses the boil.

A paste prepared by mixing equal portions of honey and white flour mixed with a little water when applied checks bleeding. The paste formed should be thick.

An immediate application of honey on the burnt area prevents the eruption of blisters.

As an expectorant:
Cough mixtures find an excellent adjunct in honey. Honey functions effectively as an expectorant. Honey and lemon juice mixed in equal quantities and melted together by gentle heating is good for the throat. For children, this mixture needs to be diluted with an equal quantity of water.

Another recipe for a home made cough syrup:

Mix one cup of honey (preferably dark honey) with one teaspoon of ginger and juice of one lemon. This mixture should be allowed to simmer for 15 minutes. For relief, one or two teaspoons of this syrup should be taken every one or two hours. Honey with hot milk is good for sore throats.

By adding one or two teaspoonful of honey to a cupful of boiling water and drinking this warm drink, refreshes and gives much relief to asthmatics.

For better complexion:
Honey taken regularly, gives a clearer complexion. A tablespoon of honey along with the juice of one medium sized lemon, taken every morning before breakfast keeps the complexion clear. It also helps in reducing weight.

For cramps:
A regular intake of honey reduces the incidence of cramps. Cramps usually occur when the calcium present in the blood is at a lower level, while the phosphorus level is high. By taking honey, the required levels are maintained in the blood.

Thus honey is a great nourisher, which besides giving energy, helps in various ways in building health.

5

Vitamins

Vitamins are organic substances essential in small quantities for normal metabolism and health. Since the body cannot manufacture vitamins, they are to be retained from food. They are also produced synthetically.

To get the best vitamin value, one should eat food in french forms. Careless cooking, over boiling of vegetables, storage in day light etc. break down the vitamins present in the food. Vitamins are classified under two group, fat soluble and water soluble.

Fat soluble vitamins are: vitamin A (retinol), vitamin D,E (tocopherol) and K. Whereas vitamin B (thiamine), B2 (riboflavin), niacin (nicotinic acid), pantothenic acid, biotin, vitamin B12, (cyanocobalamin), folic acid and vitamin C (ascorbic acid) are water soluble.

The following table will give an idea of vitamins, their functions and requirements:

Essential Vitamins

Vitamins	Best Sources	Role	RDA*
Vitamin A Retinol	Milk, butter, dark green vegetables. The body also converts pigment, carotene in yellow and green fruit and vegetable to vit. A.	Needed for body membranes such as, retina of the eye, lining of lungs and digestive system.	1mg
Thiamine B	Whole grains, enriched flour and cereals, nuts, peas, beans.	Ensures proper burning of carbohydrates.	1.0-1.4 mg.
Riboflavin (B2)	Milk and cheese.	Needed by all cells for energy release and repair.	1.2-1.7 mg.
Niacin	Whole grains, enriched flour and cereals.	Needed by cells for energy release and repair.	13-19 mg.
Pyridoxine B6	Whole grains and milk.	Needed by red blood cells and nerves for their proper functioning.	About 2mg
Pantothenic acid	Nuts and whole grains.	Needed by all cells for energy production.	4-7 mg.
Biotin	Nuts and most fresh vegetables.	Needed for skin and circulatory system.	100-200 mg
Vitamin B12	Dairy products.	Needed for red blood cells, production of bone marrow, also needed for nervous system.	3mcg
Folic acid	Fresh vegetables.	Needed for red cells production.	400 mcg.**
Vitamin C	All citrus fruits, tomatoes, raw cabbage, potatoes and strawberries.	Needed for bones, teeth and tissues for repair.	60 mg.
Vitamin D (Calciferol)	Dairy products. Some vitamins could be produced in the skin by exposing to sunlight.	Required for maintenance of blood calcium levels and thus for bone growth.	5-10 mgc.
Vitamin E	Vegetable oils and many other foods.	Needed for tissues handling fatty substances, and for formation of cell membranes.	8-10 mg.

* RDA: Recommended dietary allowances

** 'mcg' stands for microgram, which is 10^{-6} or one millionth part of a gram.

6

Minerals

Our body needs inorganic substances for forming bones, teeth and blood cells, for assisting in the chemical reactions in the blood cells and for regulating body fluids. The most important minerals which we need more than 100mg. per day are, calcium chloride, magnesium, phosphorous, potassium, sodium and sulphur. The trace elements, which we require in small quantities are: cobalt, copper, fluoride, iodine, iron, manganese, molybdenum, selenium and zinc.

How much minerals do we need?

Our body needs only a small quantity of each of the essential minerals. These minerals are not manufactured in the body and hence we need to supplement these from what we eat. The exact quantum of minerals we require is very difficult to work out, but the range of requirements mentioned below would be adequate . It is harmful to take these minerals in excess.

Minerals are not generally destroyed by cooking. The table below will give an easy reference to the various minerals, available food sources, the role they play in our body, and their daily requirement.

Essential Minerals

MINERALS	BEST SOURCES	ROLE	RDA*
Calcium	Dairy products, green vegetables	Essential for blood clotting and the structure of bones and teeth. Needed for working of nerves and all other electrically active body tissues.	About 800mg. for adults, but more during growth.
Phosphorus	Dairy products, beans and peas, cereals.	Basic cell energy store, key elements in cell reaction.	About 800mg. for adults, but more during growth.
Potassium	Avocados, bananas, apricots, potatoes, carrots, oranges, pineapple, and grapefruits.	Major minerals within body cells. Essential for fluid balance and for many cell reactions.	Not established, but what is available in fruits and vegetables is sufficient.
Magnesium	Beans and peas, nuts, cereals and green leafy vegetables.	Needed by cells, important in electrical activity of nerves and muscles.	300-350 mg.
Iodine	Iodized salt, kelp, seaweed, lettuce, pineapple juice, garlic.	Needed for thyroid gland.	About 0.1 mg.
Iron	Enriched cereals, millets, pulses, green leafy vegetables.	Needed in manufacture of Hb., the oxygen carrying compound in blood.	10-18 mg.

Fluoride, Copper, Zinc.	Water, fluoride tooth paste, whole wheat, beans, peas and nuts.	Helps to protect teeth from decay. Needed for cells to utilise oxygen. Needed in the structure of cell enzymes	About 1.5 mg. - 15 mg.
Chromium, Selenium, Molybdenum, Manganese	Trace elements available in many foods.	Minor roles in blood chemistry.	Minute amounts.
Sodium	Most foods, except fruit.	Essential for fluid balance, muscle contraction and nerve creation.	1000-3000 mg.

* RDA (Recommended dietary allowances) for non-pregnant, non-lactating adults. Please note that non-vegetarian sources are left out from best sources list.

7

Method of Cooking Food for Advantage

Cooking is an art as well as a science. Properly cooked food should be clean, hygienic, free from contaminants and at the same time preserve all nutrients, such as vitamins, minerals and other vital organic substances.

Cooking of food is primarily to improve its taste, flavour, make it easily digestible and destroy the micro-organisms present. Cooking also adds variety to the menu prepared for the family.

The cleaned and washed raw food articles are cooked with water, either by boiling or steaming, or by deep frying, seasoning, baking or grilling.

For retaining nutritive value of food the following simple rules are to be followed:

1. Wash the vegetables thoroughly before cutting.
2. Cut vegetables just before cooking and drop the cut vegetables in warm water and cook immediately.
3. Use just sufficient water for cooking.
4. Serve cooked food immediately.
5. Vegetable salads should be prepared just before serving.
6. Use acid foods such as lime juice, tomatoes, curds etc. in salads, since acid medium of raw salads prevents loss of vitamin C.

7. Fruits and vegetables should be eaten as far as possible in their natural form.
8. Soups could be prepared from the leftover water after boiling the vegetables.
9. It is better to use stainless steel vessels for cooking food.

Effect of cooking on nutritive value of food

Almost all the food we eat, except fruits and some green vegetables which are used raw in salads and chutneys, are cooked. Cooking practices, however, vary from region to region. Cooking has both advantages and disadvantages.

Effect of cooking on various nutrients:

Carbohydrates: Cooking helps in proper digestion of starch, which when cooked swells up and gets gelatinised and is digested in the body more easily.

Fat: Ordinary cooking has very little effect on fat whereas deep frying may lead to destruction of essential fatty acids and formation of toxic substances.

Proteins: Application of moderate heat splits protein and shrinks it and makes it easily digestible. But severe heat such as roasting, baking and frying reduces its nutritive value.

Vitamins: Vitamin A and D (carotene): Since these vitamins are not water soluble, no harm occurs if the water is discarded after cooking. There is very little destruction of vitamin A during cooking due to oxidation by air. Frying or roasting causes considerable loss.

Thiamine: Thiamine loss occurs during cooking due to heat, by destruction and dissolution in hot water. Loss is nearly 20-50 per cent depending on the quantity of water used for cooking.

Riboflavin (vitamin B2): Riboflavin is lost while cooking by exposure of food to strong light, by heat, discarding excess cooking water and by the addition of soda for cooking dal and vegetables. *Nicotinic acid:* Loss occurs when cooking water is discarded, and by heat during roasting and frying.

Pyridoxine: Loss occurs by destruction due to heat in cooking under pressure and by discarding excess cooking water.

Folic acid and vitamin B12: Loss of folic acid and vitamin B12 occurs by destruction due to heat in pressure cooking, roasting or frying, and by discarding excess cooking water.

Vitamin C: Loss occurs by oxidation due to exposure to air and by discarding excess cooking water. Contamination by copper also speeds up destruction of vitamin C. The quantity of vitamin C lost during cooking varies from 10-60 per cent depending upon the vegetable cooked and the method of cooking.

Minerals, calcium and phosphorous: Loss occurs when excess cooking water is discarded. When rice and dal are cooked in hard water the calcium present in the water incorporates on it.

Iron: Loss occurs when excess water is discarded. When vegetables are cut with iron knives, appreciable amount of iron incorporates on vegetables. Similarly iron percentage increases by roasting on cast-iron pans.

Sodium, potassium and magnesium: Loss occurs by leaching when excess cooking water is discarded. Sodium chloride or common salt used in cooking increases sodium content of cooked food. Increased sodium reduces potassium levels.

Effect of different methods of cooking on the nutrients present in foods:

Cooking by water, the most commonly employed method, causes moderate loss of vitamin C and slight loss of thiamine. If excess water is used and discarded, 30-70 per cent water soluble vitamins and minerals are lost.

Cooking by steam causes slight loss of vitamin C and thiamine, and negligible losses of other vitamins.

Cooking in pressure cooker results in a moderate loss of vitamin C and thiamine and slight loss of pyridoxine and vitamin B12.

Deep fat frying results in destruction of thiamine, vitamin A, carotene and vitamin C.

Shallow frying causes moderate loss of vitamin C and slight loss of vitamin A, carotene and thiamine.

27

Dry roasting leads to heavy loss of thiamine and reduces nutritive value of protein. Roasting of groundnut causes slight loss in nutritive value of protein.

Cooking soda added to cooking water causes severe loss of thiamine (70 per cent) and riboflavin (30 per cent). Addition of soda to green leafy vegetables retains colour while cooking but loss of vitamins is heavy (50-700 per cent).

Puffing of cereals and pulses causes slight loss of thiamine. Sprouting of pulses increases the vitamin C content and also the digestibility of pulse.

Cooking has several advantages as it improves the food palatability, quality and digestibility, provided it is done in limited water, steaming in pressure cookers and by following precautionary measures, then only the loss of vitamins and minerals present in it could be minimised.

8

Vegetarianism vs Non-Vegetarianism

Non-vegetarian food is still considered by majority of people as most important in the daily diet. The only good thing about non-vegetarian food is the presence of complete protein.

Due to the presence of good quantity of protein, the non-vegetarian food causes heavy work to the kidneys, which in turn lessens the efficiency of the organs leading to degenerative disorders.

Death rate among non-vegetarians by coronary heart disease is higher compared to vegetarians, because of higher levels of cholesterol and fat imbibed into the system through non-vegetarian diet.

Non-vegetarian food adds calories through the fat present in it leading to obesity, diabetes and high blood pressure. It also contains purines which produces excess uric acid in the system.

The tissues of all animals contain poisonous wastes. Hence when non-vegetarian food is consumed, toxic level in the system increases. Again, non-vegetarian food items kept in cold storage and reheated, when required, results in rapid decomposition. Since the non-vegetarian diet is relatively low in fibre content, the movement of food in the bowels slows down resulting in exposure of the large intestines to toxins present in the non-vegetarian food leading to risks of colon cancer.

Is non-vegetarian food necessary? The answer is 'no'. Although we are by nature omnivorous (capable of eating both vegetarian and non-vegetarian food), our anatomical structure - teeth, jaws, length of digestive system etc., favours diet comprising plant foods.

A well selected vegetarian diet can supply good quality protein if the following methods are followed and such food will definitely be superior to the non-vegetarian diet:

❖ By combining legumes (dried peas, beans, peanuts, etc.) with grains (barley, wheat, rice etc.)

❖ By combining legumes with nuts and seeds.

❖ Soyabean is a better substitute to meat.

9

What We Do Not Need

Coffee: A cup of coffee early in the morning, particularly in winter boosts up one's spirit. This is because the caffeine present in the coffee stimulates the adrenal gland to release adrenalin into blood stream which raises the blood sugar level, blood pressure and increases the pulse and heart rates. After a strong cup of coffee, one's performance, (both physical and mental) is at the peak. But this comes down soon and one may require another cup to boost the performance once again. This leads to addiction.

A single cup of coffee contains upto 100 mg of caffeine. Most common problems faced by coffee consumers are insomnia, slightly raised blood pressure and inability to relax.

Tea: Tea on the other hand, apart from containing tannin, (a chemical which is toxic in nature) contains caffeine to some extent.

Colas and chocolates also contain caffeine to some extent. Hence coffee, tea, colas and chocolates have to be strictly avoided during dieting periods, as they not only cause health problems but also interfere in the detoxification and cleansing process.

Alcohol: Alcoholic drinks are depressants and hence lead to severe addiction.

Alcohol consumption leads to a rise in tryglyceride (a type of fat) levels in the blood. It is also considered to be a high calorie drink (1 gm of alcohol roughly yields 7 calories, while 1 gm of fat yields 9 calories)

Severe alcohol drinking in fact leads to:

- Alcohol dependency
- Obesity
- Vitamin B deficiency
- Rise in blood pressure, with increased tendency to stroke and paralysis
- Damage of the liver
- Death, if combined with tranquilizers, sleeping pills, antihistamines and barbiturates, and
- Road accidents.

❧❧

PART II

THERAPEUTIC NUTRITION

❧❧

Introduction

Diet plays a major role in restoring the health by supplying the needed nutrients and recuperating the organs. Dieting has been advised from time immemorial, and the science of ayurveda has emphasised the importance of diet restrictions under the nomenclature "pathya" in curing the ailments. Fasting and dieting were advocated by the sages and rishis even before the advent of doctors and medical science. It was rightly said, the best doctors in the world are:

a) Doctor Diet
b) Doctor Quiet
c) Doctor Merryman.

Diet plays a unique role in curing diseases and maintaining health i.e., while sick or in healthy profile. It is the customary practice of every branch of science to involve the father of medicine, Hippocrates and his versions to support the theory and philosophy of that branch. The same is true with the naturopathy also. Hippocrates also preached "Thy food thy medicine" and "Thy medicine thy food". This great man was afflicted by migraine and followed diet restrictions for overcoming it.

But in between dietetics lost their significance and could not find a place in medical science. The doctors did not take the diet into consideration for curing or preventing diseases, and instead solely depended on medicines.

Ayurvedic system emphasises the importance of diet by saying that 'if you follow pathya, you need not take any medicine and if you do not follow the pathya, no medicine can help you'.

However, modern doctors are advocating dieting for curing disease as well as maintaining health. The patients are also increasingly following the diet to eradicate disease. It is needless to say that dieting has become popular even with people, who are figure and beauty conscious.

Therapeutical Values of Fruits and Vegetables

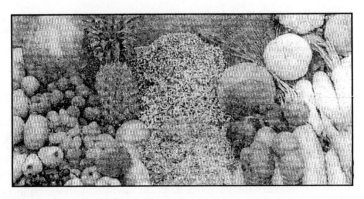

Fruits

1. *Apple:* 'An apple a day keeps the doctor away', says an old adage. Apple is the most versatile amongst all the fruits known. Its iron content is far above any other fruit. Pectin, a type of carbohydrate present in the apple, helps in stimulation and peristalsis and relieves constipation. Phosphorous contained in the fruit helps in building bones.

   Apple reduces cholesterol and is anti-oxidant. It is useful in cases of gouty, arthritis and renal stones. Apple on the whole is a food, beverage, tonic, medicine and bowel regulator.

2. *Amla:* Amla is referred to as the 'miracle fruit', immensely rich in pectin, hence very much suitable for jams, jellys,

mourabba and also for pickles. It is the richest known natural source of readily assimilated vitamin C. It can be dried and stored to make it available throughout the year. It is cooling, diuretic and laxative in nature.

To neutralise its excessive sourness, it is best combined with sweet vegetables like carrots, sweet potato, pumpkin etc. It can be used in chutneys.

3. **Banana:** It is a fruit that finds a place almost in every house in India, specially, south India. Banana should not be eaten when it is not ripe. Banana contains appreciable amounts of calcium, magnesium, phosphorous, iron and copper. It is an excellent source of vitamin C and A and a good source of vitamin B and D.

Banana soothes the stomach lining, neutralises the acid produced and also acts as an antibiotic, hence preferred in the treatment of ulcers. Banana also contains potassium, which bleaches sodium and hence is used with advantage in regulating high blood pressure.

4. *Figs:* Figs are used both in fresh and dried forms. Sugar content of dry figs is high. It is a very nourishing fruit for growing children. Figs are soaked overnight in milk or water and used. It relieves constipation.

5. *Grapes:* Red, black, purple, white, blue and green, and seeded and seedless are the varieties of grapes available in the country. It is a revitalising fruit which contains proteins, carbohydrates (grape sugar), vitamin A and B, minerals such as potassium, iron, calcium, manganese, chlorine, fluorine, sulphur and phosphorous.

The tartaric acid present in grapes stimulates liver and kidneys, and thus helps in elimination of toxins from the system. Grapes contain large amount of alkaline salts, which, when eaten in good quantities help in purifying blood as well as increasing the alkalinity of blood.

6. *Grapefruit:* It is the largest of the citrus variety fruits available. It contains more citric acid and less sugar than oranges. Popularly known as chakotha in India, it is an excellent source

of potassium and vitamin A and B. The fruit tastes bitter and hence it is advisable to eat after breakfast to stimulate appetite.

7. *Guava:* Guava is very rich in vitamin C and contains sugar. Pectin content in guava is also very high. Guava when eaten along with its seeds is highly beneficial as it regulates the bowel movement. Guava is used in making chutneys, jellys, jams and fruit cheese.

8. *Lemon:* It is a citrus fruit, rich in citric acid, and alkaline and indispensable fruit which is useful in many ways. The juice of lime when added to almost all recipes enhances flavour and taste. Lemon is also used for making pickles. Common misconception regarding lemon is that it tends to increase the acidity, but on the contrary the lime juice converts itself into an alkaline ash after complete digestion.

   Lime juice with honey or salt in the morning on an empty stomach is good since it helps to maintain the alkalinity of blood and also purifies it. It is ideal for people suffering from arthritis, because the vitamin C in lime juice strengthens connective tissues of the joints. It also improves the vitality and hence is very useful in treating causes of cold, running nose, cough and other acute conditions.

9. *Mango:* Delicious and a great nourisher of the body, it is available in umpteen varieties from May to August. Mangoes are consumed in various forms. It can be eaten directly, made into a juice, added to rice dishes and sweets and as milk shake. It is always easily digestible.

   Raw unripe mango finds its use in making pickles, chutneys and salads.

   Mango is rich in vitamin A and C. People with diabetes and obesity should not eat mangoes too often.

10. *Watermelon(Tarbuza):* A fruit with full of water and is excellent to quench thirst during summer, and being low in calories it is ideal for weight watchers. It is cooling, refreshing and also rich in vitamin C.

11. *Muskmelon (Kharbuze):* It is rich in alkaline salts, beneficial in treatment of hyperacidity, ulcers and other digestive

39

disorders. The pulp, generally mashed, mixed with water and jaggery is an excellent drink during summer to quench thirst.

12. *Orange:* It is one of the citrus variety of fruits rich in vitamin A,B and C and calcium. It is highly beneficial for digestive disorders. It is an excellent blood purifier. Oranges eaten as it is or made into a juice or marmalade is very nourishing.

13. *Papaya:* A very useful fruit available all through the year is indispensable to mankind for its medicinal properties. It is the only fruit which, perhaps can be eaten by everybody without any harm.

Easily digestible due to the enzyme papaine, chymopapaine present in papaya is almost similar to enzyme secreted in stomach called pepsin.

Papaya is highly alkaline and helps in maintaining alkaline balance of the body. It is very rich in vitamin A,B,C and D, apart from certain other essential minerals such as calcium, phosphorous and iron. Papaya is highly beneficial in digestive disorders, constipation, renal stone and other disorders. Raw papaya can be used as a vegetable.

14. *Pomegranate:* Pomegranate is rich in sugar, iron and citric acid. It is highly nutritious and delicious. Pomegranate with seeds is good for people suffering from constipation and its juice prevents diarrhoea.

15. *Pineapple:* A very delicious fruit with good medicinal properties. Pineapple juice helps in digestion due to the presence of a substance, which is almost similar to pepsin present in the stomach.

It raises alkalinity of blood, is a powerful blood purifier, useful in acidosis, gouty and rheumatoid arthritis. It also helps in removing excess water, thus relieving oedema and swellings of the body.

Pineapple cannot be cut and eaten with its rough skin as it often produces irritation in the throat. But it should not be avoided just for that reason, as it is an ideal fruit for patients suffering from asthma and bronchitis.

16. *Passion fruit:* It is another citrus variety fruit similar to lemon and can be substituted for lemon juice. The advantage of passion

fruit juice over lemon is its appealing colour and flavour. Passion fruit juice is a good source of vitamin A.

17. **Peaches:** These are sub-acid fruits. It is a juicy fruit containing 80 per cent moisture. It is a good source of iron and potassium.

18. **Pear:** It is popularly known as *naspathi* in Hindi. It is also a sub-acid fruit related to apple, but contains more sugar and less acid. It is useful in cases of bladder stones.

19. **Sapota (cheeku):** Sweetest of all the fruits containing high percentage of sugar. It is a high calorie fruit and hence diabetes and obesity patients should avoid it. Sapota contains good amount of fibre and is useful in relieving constipation. It is also ideally suited for treating digestive disorders, especially hyperacidity, ulcers, colitis, dysentry etc.

20. **Custard Apple (seethaphal):** It is another sweet fruit high in calories and should be avoided by diabetics and obese patients. It is soft, easily digestible and ideally suited for ulcer and hyperacidity patients. It is a good source of iron and vitamin C.

Dry fruits

When the moisture present in a fruit evaporates it forms a dry fruit. By drying the fruit it can be made available throughout the year. When soaked in water they almost retain their original fresh fruit form.

Generally available dry fruits are: dry figs, raisins, prunes, dates and apricots.

1. **Dates:** Delicious, sweet dried fruit and can be eaten as it is. It is also often used as a sweetener substituting sugar or jaggery. Dates contain very high percentage of sugar, fair amount of protein and is an excellent source of iron. Dates and milk are ideal for improving health and nourishment. Dates soaked in milk or water overnight and taken next day helps in bowel movements. It is an ideal nourisher for children, emaciated and aged people.

2. **Figs:** Dried fig is very rich in sugar, calcium and protein. It is most effective in relieving constipation, when soaked in milk overnight and taken the next day. It is a healthy food and highly nutritious.

41

3. **Prunes:** These must be avoided by patients suffering from gouty, arthritis, high uric acid and renal calculi patients, as they contain high levels of benzoic acid, which leads to acidosis.

It is also useful in relieving constipation, when used by soaking it overnight in milk or water.

4. **Raisins:** Raisins are highly alkaline and are excellent blood purifiers. Raisins contain good amount of calcium, phosphorous and iron. Raisins are often used in making sweets, are also very useful in relieving constipation.

Vegetables

Vegetables are consumed in the form of leaf, stem, root, shoot and flower. They are either used raw or after cooking.

Amaranthus: A commonly used leafy vegetable in South India and is a good source of calcium, iron, vitamin A and C and folic acid. It not only provides nourishment, but also helps in regulating the bowel because of the presence of fibre.

Agathi(agasthi): Another leafy vegetable used in southern parts of India. An excellent source of iron and calcium and good source of protein, vitamin A and C.

Cabbage: Cabbage is considered highly useful because of its high mineral and vitamin content and alkaline salts present in it. Cabbage is a good source of vitamin C. For best results, cabbage should be eaten raw. It also contains a good amount of sulphur, lime and iron. Cabbage gives a strange odour when cooked. Recent researches have identified in it a substance which has certain qualities in healing ulcers of stomach. Hence it is advisable to take it in cooked form in all digestive disorders.

Celery leaves: Celery's edible portions are stalk, leaf and root. It is a good source of iron, calcium, phosphorous, vitamin A and C and protein. Celery is a diuretic and good for diabetics and obese patients. It is an excellent carminative and helps in bowel regulation. Celery and carrot juice is an excellent combination.

Chekkur manis: Is a plant of Malaysia, now popular in Kerala and Karnataka. It is otherwise known as multivitamin plant. It is a good source of calcium, phosphorous, iron, protein and vitamin A, and C.

Coriander leaves: This leafy vegetable is extensively used in garnishing vegetables, cereal preparations and salads. It enhances flavour and taste of the recipe when added. It is an excellent source of calcium, phosphorous, iron, potassium and vitamin A, Bl, B2, and niacin (since it contains good amount of iron, it is good for anaemic patients). The juice of coriander leaves mixed with 1 teaspoon of honey and taken 2-3 times a day improves anaemic conditions.

Curry leaves: Another leafy vegetable mostly used in dishes for seasoning, that enhances the flavour and taste of the recipe. It is also used in making chutney powder and chutney. It is highly nutritious and an excellent source of calcium, phosphorous, iron, protein and vitamin A, B1,B2, niacin and C.

Curry leaf is very good in curing digestive disorders. It also finds its use in treating diabetes.

Methi leaves (fenugreek leaves): A very popular vegetable used in India to make vegetable dishes, rice dishes, to stuff in chapatis, paranthas etc. Methi is used to stimulate scalp. Soaking methi seeds overnight, grinding it to a paste, applying it on scalp for an hour and washing it off, cools the scalp and helps in preventing dandruff formation. Methi is an excellent source of iron, protein, calcium, vitamin A, B1 and B2. Methi seeds soaked overnight in curds and consumed is an excellent measure to control sugar levels in a diabetic patient.

Drumstick leaves: Used in making vegetable dishes. Flowers of the tree are also used in recipes. Drumstick leaves are an excellent source of calcium, magnesium, phosphorous, protein and vitamins such as A, thiamine, B2 and C.

Spinach: A very popular leafy vegetable used in India. It is used in making vegetable preparations, dal, rice dishes, in salads, soups etc.

Spinach is very nutritive and ideal for children, pregnant and lactating mothers. It is an excellent source of iron and vitamin A and C. It is a good source of protein, fibre, calcium, phosphorous, thiamine and riboflavin.

Lettuce: Though lettuce contains a good amount of iron, most of it is lost when cooked. Hence lettuce is generally used for making salads. In the salad form it is very useful to children, pregnant and lactating mothers. Besides iron, lettuce is an excellent source of folic acid. Hence it is useful in removing iron deficiency as well as folic acid deficiency anaemia.

It is also a good source for other nutrients such as calcium, potassium, vitamin A and B2.

Mint: Popularly known as pudina, it is used for making chutneys, soups, sauces, drinks, in vegetables, and rice dishes for garnishing and in salads. Mint is carminative hence very useful in digestive disorders such as gas trouble, flatulence and indigestion.

Mint is an excellent source of iron and protein, good source of calcium, phosphorous, vitamin-thiamin, B2, niacin, C and A.

Roots and tubers

This class of vegetables are rich in carbohydrates, low in fat and protein. Important roots and tubers mainly used in India are: beetroot, carrot, potato, sweet potato, radish, turnip etc.

1. *Beetroot:* Beetroots are juicy and rich in alkaline salts. Main substance is sugar and not starch. It is used by baking, boiling or steaming. It is used as a vegetable dish and in making sweet dish called beetroot halwa. It is a good source of potassium, sodium, magnesium and iron.

2. *Radish:* Another juicy root vegetable which has a pungent flavour. It is eaten raw in combination with other vegetables or in cooked form. Radish is used for making chutneys also. A very low calorie vegetable, it has a diuretic effect hence preferred in cases of renal stones

3. *Turnip:* This root vegetable contains less sugar than beetroot, or carrots. It is a rich source of calcium.

4. *Carrot:* Carrot is a versatile root vegetable, which is consumed both in raw and cooked form. Carrot contains a yellow pigment called carotene, a pro-vitamin which later converts itself into vitamin A. The carotene gives good colour to the skin. Carrot is an excellent source of phosphorous, carotene (vitamin A), folic acid, sodium, potassium and vitamin C. It is very effective

in correcting night blindness (vitamin A deficiency), anaemia, acidosis and is a good blood purifier.

Carrot and celery juice is an excellent combination for treating arthritis. Carrots should never be washed after peeling to retain its nutritive value.

Carrot juice is a great nourisher for asthmatics, hyperacidity, ulcer and undernourished patients.

5. *Potato:* It is a staple food in India. It is almost equal to cereals as far as its nutritive value is concerned. Potato contains starch which is easily digestible. Unlike other cereals, potato is alkaline in nature.

   Potato consists of approximately 70 per cent moisture, 20 per cent carbohydrates, 2 per cent protein, and minerals such as potassium and magnesium. It is a good source of vitamin C. Potato has to be eaten with its skin intact to preserve its nutritive value. It is an excellent low cost substitute for cereals. A baked potato or cooked potato is ideal for children as a breakfast dish.

6. *Sweet potato:* It is similar to potato as far as the sweetness is concerned. Sugar in sweet potato is slightly more than that of the white potato. Sweet potato can be used raw or cooked. It is used for stuffing in parathas or used as a vegetable dish. It is also used to make sweet dishes like halwa and poli (South Indian delicacy). Sweet potato is a good source of vitamin C, minerals such as magnesium, calcium and potassium.

7. *Onion:* A root vegetable classified under spice category and is extensively used all over India. Onion is used almost in every edible vegetable dish, chapati, chutney, sambar, soup, salad, or even a chat. Onion when cut gives a characteristic strong odour. Onion has medicinal values also. Smell of onion when inhaled opens up the blocked nostrils.

   It is a good stimulant, hence very ideal for use in all digestive disorders. Onion oxidises cholesterol, hence reduces cholesterol levels. One teaspoon of raw onion juice on rising from bed is good for reducing cholesterol.

   Finely chopped onions mixed in honey kept for a day and used 2-3 tsp/day is an excellent medicine for asthmatics.

Onion is carminative, diuretic, stimulant and anti-inflammatory. Onion is also a powerful antiseptic, attracts germs and poisons, and can be used with advantage in treating wounds.

Onion contains at least 80 per cent moisture. It is a good source of vitamin C, organic salts like calcium, potassium, iron, phosphorous, magnesium and sulphur.

8. *Garlic:* It is a nature's gift, having remarkable curative properties. Being a germicidal and a blood purifier, it is very useful in treating intestinal problems and also to replace intestinal flora. It is very effective in bringing down cholesterol, hence it is used for preventing heart diseases. It also helps in relieving flatulence gas from the stomach.

Garlic is a good source of phosphorous, zinc, potassium and iodine.

9. *Ginger:* Another root, classified under spices, is also used extensively in preparation of eatables. Ginger also possesses certain therapeutic properties.

It contains 80 per cent moisture, little amount of protein and fibre. It is a good source of iron, magnesium, manganese and zinc.

Ginger is used in almost all good preparations to enhance flavour and taste. Ginger is also carminative, stimulant and blood purifier. It stimulates appetite. A teaspoon full of ginger juice mixed with a teaspoon full of honey in warm water is a good remedy for asthmatics.

Other vegetables

10. *Gourd variety vegetables:* Vegetables such as ashgourd, bitter gourd, bottle gourd, snake gourd and ridged gourd are generally watery vegetables containing at least 80-90 per cent moisture. As they are low in calories they are ideal to satisfy hunger without adding more calories, hence good for people who desire to lose weight and are diabetics. These are also good sources of vitamin C and minerals such as potassium, magnesium and sodium.

11. *French beans:* This vegetable comes under high calorie vegetable, which contains a little amount of protein. It is a

good source of folic acid, vitamin C and minerals such as magnesium, potassium, sulphur and zinc.

12. **Cauliflower:** It is another low calorie vegetable which contains 90 per cent moisture and some amount of protein. It is a good source of phosphorous, iron, potassium, sulphur and zinc.

13. **Knol Khol:** Its moisture content being 93 per cent is ideal for diabetics and obese patients. It is a good source of iron, sodium, sulphur, chloride and vitamin C.

14. **Cucumber:** It is a highly alkaline food and a good source of vitamin A and C. Moisture content being 97 per cent, ideal for eating to satisfy appetite and hence beneficial for diabetics and obese patients.

    It is mainly used in salads and to make health drinks. Since it has diuretic properties, it is useful for people with urinary problems. It is cooling in effect and is of immense use to quench thirst during hot summer.

15. **Capsicum:** Pungent vegetable and is a powerful stimulant. In spite of being pungent, it does not irritate, like the green chilli, the soft internal lining of the digestive system. Capsicum is used raw in salads, raithas and cooked and used as a vegetable. Capsicum contains 93 per cent moisture and is a good source of magnesium and vitamin C.

16. **Bangalore brinjal:** It is extensively used in Karnataka for making dal, chutney and vegetable dishes. Its moisture content is roughly about 93 per cent and is a good source of calcium. Being a low calorie vegetable, ideal for obese patients, diabetics and asthmatics.

17. **Kundri:** Another low calorie tasty vegetable, even if it is eaten raw. It contains 94 per cent moisture and is a good source of folic acid, vitamin C and magnesium.

18. **Lady's finger:** It is a vegetable which contains good amount of fibre and is very good for bowel regulation. It is an excellent source of folic acid, phosphorous, magnesium, potassium, sulphur and chloride.

19. **Tinda:** Another low calorie vegetable which contains at least 94 per cent moisture, and a good source of vitamin C, sodium and chloride.

47

20. *Tomato:* Tomato is both used as a fruit as well as a vegetable and can be used in almost every eatable. Tomato is used raw in salads, for garnishing in chats, used in making raitas, chutneys, sauces and soups. It is also used in dal, sambar and in vegetable and rice preparations. Tomato when ripe is actually a sub-acid fruit.

Tomato is an excellent source of iron, potassium, sodium, sulphur, chloride and vitamin C.

The belief that tomatoes are harmful for people with high uric acid, gout and rheumatism is probably because of oxalic acid and citric acid present in it. But going by the amount of oxalic acid it contains, one need not restrict taking tomato in all forms of arthritis.

Food leaving acid (Acidic foods)

The end product of the following foods is acidic.

All non-vegetarian food/s

Cereals	-	refined wheat, barley, polished rice, corn, white bread, cakes, pastries and biscuits.
Fruits	-	unripe banana, plums and prunes.
Vegetables	-	beans, peas and rhubarb.
Cheese	-	processed chocolate, coffee, tea, grain, lentils and sugar.

Foods leaving alkaline (Alkaline foods)

The end product of the following foods is alkaline.

Cereals	-	unpolished rice, whole wheat and ragi.
Fruits	-	apple, apricots, fully ripened banana, berries, cherries, dates, figs(fresh), figs (dry), grapes, grapefruit, lemons, melons, oranges, peaches, pears, pineapples, raisins, almonds.
Vegetables	-	beetroot, cabbage, carrot, celery, cauliflower, cucumber, lettuce, parsley, potato, pumpkin, radish, spinach, tomato, turnip, onion, cottage cheese and soyabean.

Respiratory Disorders and Diet

The oxygen we breathe in passes through bronchial tubes and lungs to different parts of the body via blood. Similarly, the carbon dioxide in the impure blood is breathed out after passing through the lungs and bronchial tubes.

The impurities in the blood are brought to the lungs for final disposal in the form of expectoration. The soft mucosal inner lining of the lungs is constantly exposed to such impurities and are cast off producing a thick substance called phlegm.

The respiratory system throws out this unwanted mucus through cold, running nose, sneezing and cough.

Since the blood will be continuously bringing all kinds of impurities to lungs, most often the respiratory system becomes the seat of many diseases. Due to irregular eating habits, the morbid matter starts accumulating in the tissues of the respiratory system and the diseases causing micro-organisms, inhaled during respiration starts multiplying causing upper respiratory infections. Antibiotics taken suppress the bacterial activity temporarily, but lower one's vitality.

In the present day world due to wrong eating habits and polluted atmosphere, the respiratory diseases are becoming common. Lack of exercise, wearing of too much of protective garments leading to reduction in skin activity, and the inability to use the lungs to their full capacity in breathing are the other factors contributing to the increased incidence of respiratory diseases.

The significant indicators of respiratory diseases are: cold, running nose, sneezing and accumulation of secretions in the sinuses leading to sinusitis. The accumulation of secretions inside the lungs leads to cough, breathing difficulty etc.

The manifestation of symptoms are nothing but the healing efforts of the body and a warning signal to an individual that something has gone wrong in the system. If the individual recognises it and rectifies the wrong eating habits and alters the other factors responsible for respiratory illness, half the battle is actually won and the rest 'mother nature' will take care. A few simple measures regarding diet are suggested below to overcome common respiratory ailments.

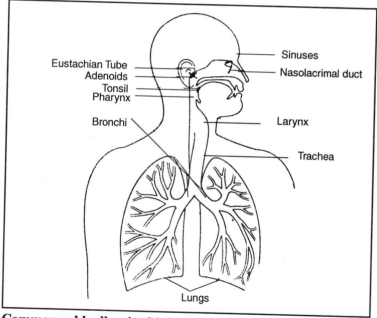

Common cold, allergic rhinitis, sinusitis etc.:

✧ Fasting for 2-3 days or till symptoms persist on juices specially citrus fruit juices. (Fasting, however, should be undertaken under the supervision of an expert).

✧ Plenty of warm liquids and soups should be taken as these relieves congestion.

✧ After breaking the fast, eating habits have to be corrected avoiding tea, coffee, use of milk and milk products and fruits such as, banana.

✧ Eating too much of sugary products and starches and non-vegetarian food, cold foods, sweets, ice-creams etc. should also be avoided.

✧ Yogic kriyas, pranayama and asana play a vital role in curing respiratory diseases.

Acute and chronic bronchitis, bronchial asthma:

✧ All the above measures adopted to treat common cold.

✧ Citrus fruits should be avoided. When cough persists in the case of typical asthma attack, fruits like oranges and pineapple and lemon juice should be avoided and instead, softer variety of fruits like sapota, papaya, apples, watermelon etc., can be taken. Banana should be totally restricted.

✧ An asthmatic should not fill the stomach fully as the pressure built up in the stomach presses the lungs leading to aggravation of the condition.

✧ Care should be taken by avoiding the gas forming foods so that gastritis could be taken care off. Gastritis leads to bronchitis.

✧ Milk and milk products cause phelgm formation leading to congestion in the lungs. Hence these should be avoided.

✧ Avoid foods which cause constipation. The hardness and congestion of intestine increase pressure in abdomen and cause negative pressure in the lungs, which prevents their full expansion.

✧ The good amount of fruits and vegetables having high fibre content should be consumed.

✧ Avoid deep fried foods, which are hard to digest.

✧ Early dinner is best suited for patients of respiratory ailment. It ensures complete digestion before retirement.

✧ Hot honey water (one teaspoon honey + one glass of water) before bed relaxes the throat by clearing accumulated phlegm in the throat.

✧ Take plenty of soup.

✧ Avoid white sugar completely and use jaggery.

✧ Take alkaline foods with 70 per cent vegetables, salad, fru
  soups and 30 per cent cereals like rice, wheat, ragi, jawa

✧ Avoid rice, at dinner.

✧ Avoid cold foods, ice creams, soft drinks and frozen foods and
  drinks.

A typical menu for bronchial asthma patients:

6.30 am	-	A glass of hot *Tulsi* water with honey and ginger.
8.00 am	-	A fruit and soup/fruit juice/carrot juice.
11.00 am	-	300 gms boiled vegetables.
to		200 gms rice/3 chapaties/200 gms vegetable dalia
1.00 pm		Alternate days dal/soup.
Afternoon	-	Fruit juice/carrot juice.
Dinner	-	2 or 3 fruits, steamed vegetables, sprouts and soup.
(6pm-7pm)		
Night	-	A glass of hot *Tulsi* water with honey and ginger
(9-10pm)		as and when required.

Hypertension

Hypertension is a disease of the modern society. The people living in urban and semi-urban areas of industrially developed countries are more prone to this problem than people in the rural areas.

Hypertension strikes an individual without giving any indication, hence, it is termed as a 'silent killer'.

Since the definite cause for hypertension is not known, the disease could be controlled by taking care of the risk factors such as:

a) Wrong eating habits.

b) Smoking and alcohol.

c) Excess salt intake.

d) Lack of exercise.

e) Physical and mental stress.

f) Obesity.

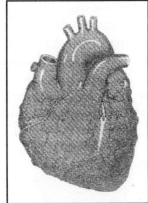

One should try to maintain the blood pressure within the safe range of 110/70 - 130/80 mm/hg.

Diet plays a very important role in the maintenance of blood pressure by influencing the quality of blood flowing in the arterial stream.

The hypertensive should take the following precautions for the diet:

- Calories should be restricted, if one is overweight.
- Diet should be low in cholesterol and maximum allowable cholesterol is 300 mg per day.
- Diet should be free from saturated fatty acids. Instead, polyunsaturated fatty acids are to be preferred.
- Fatty foods such as oil, butter, ghee, etc. should be restricted to 2-3 tbsp a day.
- Dietary fibre should be increased.
- All fried foods, sweets, sugary foods such as jams, marmalades, pastries, cakes etc., should be avoided.
- All salted nuts, salted chips, pickles, preserved foods should be avoided.
- At least 8-10 glasses of water should be drunk daily.
- Salt should be restricted to 1 gm/day.
- More fruits which are rich in potassium, such as sweetlime (*mosambi*), orange, muskmelon (*tarbuj*), peaches, plums and sapota should be taken.
- Natural diuretics like tender coconut water, barley water, butter-milk, dhania water can be taken to increase urine output and to reduce high BP.
- If the patient is diabetic, care should be taken that the blood sugar level should not exceed the normal levels.
- Eat plenty of raw salads, fruits and vegetables to maintain the consistency of blood in order to flow easily in the vessels.
- Avoid salt while cooking vegetables. Use salt on the table.
- Rest, relaxation and sound sleep are effective factors to keep the BP under control.

Diabetes Mellitus

Diabetes mellitus like hypertension is a disease of modern civilisation. The kind of lifestyle people lead - such as wrong eating habits, lack of exercise, habits such as tea, coffee and drinking alcohol, smoking, stress and strain are all linked to high prevalence of diabetes. But, the disease is more common in urban areas because of these 'urban' habits than in rural areas where life is quieter.

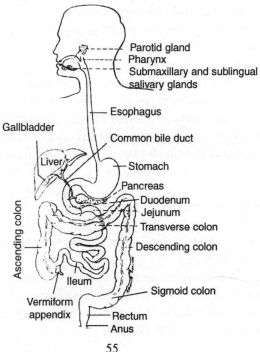

Management of diabetes

Most of the non-insulin dependent diabetes could be treated through diet, nature cure treatments, yoga, physical exercise and relaxation. The purpose of treatment is to keep the levels of blood sugar within the safe limits (fasting blood sugar upto 100 mg, post-lunch blood sugar 140 mg). In addition, educating a diabetic is also important because it is a condition to be treated through a diet. (Photo liver and pancreas)

Diet

Diet of a diabetic is in no way different from that of a normal man. When a normal person eats, pancreas in his body automatically releases the required quantity of insulin to maintain normal sugar level. But in a diabetic this mechanism would be either defective or less efficient. Hence a diabetic should take care of the quantity and the type of food he/she takes in order to maintain sugar levels within normal range.

* ❖ A diabetic diet should consist of 60-70 per cent of carbohydrates, particularly complex carbohydrates, 15-20 per cent fats and 15-20 per cent proteins.
* ❖ Fat intake is to be restricted and polyunsaturated fatty acids should be preferred to saturated fats.
* ❖ Food rich in fibre should be preferred.
* ❖ Daily intake of calories should be restricted.
* ❖ Pulses and dals are the only sources of proteins in the vegetarian diet. Hence, diabetics should use them moderately.
* ❖ Non-vegetarian food should be strictly avoided.
* ❖ Milk intake should also be restricted to minimum.
* ❖ Milk products, such as buttermilk and curds should be used in plenty.
* ❖ Nuts should be restricted to minimum.
* ❖ Vegetables and greens contain a lot of fibre, vitamins and minerals and have low calorific value and hence they should be used in plenty.
* ❖ Fruits contain some quantity of sugar, moisture, minerals and vitamins. Fruits like banana, seedless grapes, sapota (*cheeku*), leechi, jackfruit, custard apple (*sharifa*), mango, and dry fruits like raisins should be avoided.

- Unsweetened fruit juices, lime juice, soups and salads should be used in plenty.
- Sweets, sugar, glucose, sugary products like jams, marmalades, jellys, ice-creams and desserts should be avoided strictly.
- Use of jaggery or honey is to be restricted to 2-3 teaspoons a day.
- Beverages such as coffee, tea, bournvita, horlicks, colas and alcohol should be strictly avoided.
- Refined foods made of maida, such as whitebread, biscuits, cakes and pastries should be avoided. Instead wheat, sooji and bread can be used.
- Cough syrups which contain sugar, diuretics which reduce glucose tolerance, steroids reducing the action of insulin, and betablockers are to be used with caution.
- At least 8-10 glasses of water should be taken per day.
- Chewing *Tulsi* leaves daily is also found to be beneficial.

The following vegetables and fruits are to be used sparingly and with caution: potato, carrot, beetroot, tapioca, peas, beans, sweet potato and cluster beans.

A Typical diabetic diet

6.60 am	- A glass of curd methi. (About 1 tsp of methi seeds soaked in curds overnight)
8.00 am	- One kind of fruit, raw salad and a cup of buttermilk.
11.00 am	- Tender coconut water.
1.00 pm	- 100 gms of salads.
	- 200 gms of boiled vegetables.
(Lunch)	- 3 chapatis/200 gms rice/a medium sized ragi ball. 300 gms veg. dalia. Every alternate day 1 cup of dal. Buttermilk/soup.
4.00 pm	- a glass of buttermilk/unsweetened fruit juice.
6.00 pm	- 2 or 3 varieties of fruits (only fruits allowed),
7.00 pm	Steamed vegetables, sprouts and soup/buttermilk
	OR
	Cooked food as mentioned for lunch, if one feels week. (No salads and rice)
8.00 pm	- a glass of skimmed milk/buttermilk (if necessary).

Musculoskeletal Disorders

Arthritis

Arthritis is a disease of the modern times and prevalent everywhere. Habits such as improper eating, sedentary lifestyle, stress and strain will have an impact on the joints leading to different types of arthritis.

The moment one comes to know that one is suffering from arthritis, one tends to imagine to be crippled within no time and this fear and frustration leads to loss of confidence giving room for further advancement of the disease.

Osteoarthritis

This is the most common type of degenerative joint disorder, which generally affects the knees, hips, ankles and spinal cord and rarely the shoulder joints.

An osteoarthritis patient is usually a middle aged, overweight individual. Hence reducing weight is mandatory, if the person is obese.

Rheumatoid arthritis

It is a crippling disease and may progress faster and damage the joints. Most of the rheumatoid arthritis victims would be of 20-40 age group. This will cause pain and stiffness specially in the small joints, fingers, wrists, elbows, knees and ankles. Many long suffering arthritis patients develop crippling deformities of hands and feet limiting their movements.

Gouty arthritis

Generally gouty arthritis patients will be in good health. But at times it causes a severe pain in the great toe and the severity would be so great that even at the slightest touch one withdraws the toe. It is generally the great toe, rarely ankles and knees, that suffers from the disease. Most of the gouty arthritis patients get such episodic attacks periodically in the first year and once in a while thereafter.

Ankylosing spondylitis

Generally affects those aged above 40 with restricted movements around the spinal cord either at the neck or lower back.

Cervical and lumbar spondylitis

This is another commonly occurring degenerative type of arthritis affecting cervical and lumbar regions. Almost all forms of arthritis can be treated with diet, exercises, hydrotherapy and physiotherapy.

Diet plays a very important role in the treatment. The synovial fluid, which bathes all the movable joints consists of water, minerals and microprotein derived from the food we eat.

Excessive intake of protein is also not good as the nitrogen content in the excess protein gets accumulated and causes muscular fatigue, increased blood urea and uric acid (since these two are the end products of protein metabolism) and the gouty arthritis is solely due to increased uric acid level. Also, excess protein in blood causes sticky nature in red blood cells leading to inflammation of joints and a raised ESR level.

Fat and sat are the primary causes of almost all forms of arthritis with fat as a major factor. When the fat level increases in the blood stream, it pools the red blood cells restricting the blood flow through the blood vessels. This restricted blood flow leads to reduced oxygen levels, indirectly destroying the cells of immune system, and leakage of some powerful enzymes into the joints, which will lead to rheumatoid arthritis. Salt retains water and the accumulated water soon floods the tissues around the joints, further restricting the blood flow.

Food allergy plays a great role in rheumatoid arthritis. Eighty per cent of the people with rheumatoid arthritis are allergic to certain foods. Rheumatoid arthritis is also otherwise known as autoimmune disorder. Allergic reactions generally are aggravation of swelling, redness, pain and inflammation, limiting the joint movements. Food allergy is a known cause for rheumatoid arthritis, but which type of food acts as an allergen is, in fact, difficult to find out.

It is advisable for all rheumatoid arthritis sufferers to make a list of all things and events which aggravate the symptoms so that they could be avoided.

Diet is very important in the treatment of all forms of arthritis. Careful monitoring of diet and elimination of such food items which aggravate the symptoms is needed so that they could be avoided.

Diet is very important in the treatment of all forms of arthritis. Careful monitoring of diet and elimination of such food items which aggravate the condition and adjusting of food to individual needs will go a long way in the treatment of arthritis.

Do's and dont's about the diet for arthritis:

- ◆ Fast, to start with, 2-3 days under medical supervision in an institutional set-up.
- ◆ Diet of an arthritic patient should be low in fat, protein and salt.
- ◆ Avoid milk, curds and buttermilk.
- ◆ Avoid fried foods, butter, processed cheese, whole milk, non-vegetarian food, most of the nuts and seeds, cakes, pastries and refined sugar
- ◆ Stop alcohol, coffee, tea and smoking.
- ◆ Take sparingly skimmed milk, cereals, grains, fruits and vegetable salads.
- ◆ Weight reduction is mandatory for the overweight arthritic patient. Avoid extra load on the weight bearing joints, specially lower back, hip, knee and ankle joints.
- ◆ Foods containing high protein content, specially non-vegetarian food, asparagus, spinach, mushrooms, cauliflower, lentils and pea etc., should be restricted specially in case of gouty arthritis cases (Table of protein content of various foods is given at the end of this book).

◆ Take plenty of citrus fruits and fruit juices which contain vitamin 'C', which not only improves immunity but also strengthens collagen, a prateriol which protects the joint and connective tissues. A popular misconception among people is that citrus fruits increase acidity, but on the contrary the acids present in citrus fruits give rise to alkaline ash at the end of metabolism.

◆ An arthritic should be encouraged to eat plenty of fruits, vegetables, and salads, which not only increase alkalinity of blood but are also rich in potassium, a mineral which helps in removing excess body fluid due to excess consumption of salt.

Disorders of the Digestive System

'A healthy stomach is a healthy body' says an old adage. More than 60 per cent of all the diseases have their roots in the digestive system. Unlike other fatal diseases such as hypertension, heart attack, cancer etc., digestive disorders are not a threat to life, and we often ignore them.

Broadly speaking most of the digestive disorders are due to:
   i) Improper eating habits, such as irregular meal timings, heavy and excess late night dinners, junk foods, eating very spicy food and drinking too much of coffee, tea, alcohol and smoking.
  ii) Stress and strain, physical as well as mental state of a person are equally important
 iii) Over medication with pain killers like aspirin, non-steroid anti-inflammatory drugs, cortisones and other medicines on empty stomach.

Diet during indigestion, gas trouble, dyspepsia and reflux oesophagitis

Indigestion is the commonest problem many people often suffer from. They attribute the indigestion to overeating, but in addition to overeating, the type and quality of food also play a role in causing indigestion.

The combination of fried food, sweets, sugar, starch and above all, drinking liquids in between causes bloating of stomach and the volatile fatty acids present in the food float at the top and hence most of the time oily smell is felt in the throat during belching, particularly after a rich meal.

Irregular meal habits not only kill normal response of the body to food, but also disturb the secretions of gastric juice.

Indigestion leads to unpleasant bloated sensation in the stomach leading to pain in the abdomen and sometimes food regurgitates back into the foodpipe, and this condition is known as reflux oesophagitis.

Dietary precautions:

- Fasting on suitable liquids for 3/4 days can take care of indigestion.
- Food should be simple consisting of cereals, fruits, vegetables, salads and soups.
- Avoid fried foods, sweets and drinking liquids inbetween, while eating.
- Get up from the dining table even when you have a feeling that you could eat some more.
- Avoid raw cucumber, radish, carrots, and raw chutneys.
- Avoid stale (previous night leftovers) food.
- Eating too much of vegetables and foods like beans, milk, pastries, chocolates and carbonated drinks must be avoided.
- Chewing of food thoroughly is very important
- Hurry, worry and anxiety must be avoided while eating.

Hyperacidity and heartburn

Stomach produces hydrochloric acid, which not only acts as a protective barrier to the mucosal lining of abdomen but also helps digestion. But when there is over production of the acid it results in burning sensation in the chest area which is called "heartburn". Untreated hyperacidity leads to peptic ulcers.

Increased intra-abdominal pressure in cases of obesity and pregnancy also leads to heartburn sometimes.

Dietary precautions:

- Drink 2/3 glasses of cold water soon after getting up from bed early in the morning. It dilutes and washes away the acid secretion of overnight.
- Take small meals at frequent intervals i.e., 3-4 hours once.
- Take cold milk whenever acidity persists.
- Tea, coffee, smoking, alcohol and spicy food should be strictly avoided.
- Reduction of weight lessens intra-abdominal pressure and hence, is very important.
- Avoid lying down immediately after taking food.
- Avoid hot food and hot liquids.
- Avoid white sugar strictly as it enhances acidity by increasing fermentation. Use jaggery instead.
- Take measures to avoid constipation.
- Drink at least 8-12 glasses of water in a day.
- Avoid spicy, irritant foods.
- Take bland diet with minimum salt, as salt is also an irritant.
- Take plenty of natural antacids like coconut water, sweet buttermilk, cold milk and ashgourd juice.
- The chlorophyll present in green leafy vegetable is also an excellent agent to neutralise acidity.
- Avoid sour fruits, if not suitable.

Gastritis

Bloated sensation in the abdomen after eating, belching, heartburn, pain in the upper abdominal region and general weakness are characteristic features of gastritis. It is due to severe inflammation of gastric mucosa (inner lining of stomach). Symptoms of gastritis are vomiting of partly digested food, headache, fever, diarrhoea and constipation.

Dietary precautions:

- Nothing should be consumed, except ice cold milk at regular intervals till symptoms subside.
- Once the symptoms subside, small meals consisting of meshy fruits at regular interval (once in every 2 hrs) should be taken.

- Hot liquids and hot food should be avoided.
- Fried foods, tea, coffee, alcohol, citrus fruits and fruit juices should be completely avoided.
- Plenty of non-fat buttermilk and curds should be taken.
- Pain killers, anti-inflammatory and steroid drugs should be totally discontinued.

Peptic ulcer

Ulcer is the discontinuity of the mucus membrane of the stomach. The excess acid produced in the stomach burns the mucus membrane exposing the raw inflamed area. Whenever the acid flows down on that area, it causes burning sensation followed by pain, which subsides after taking cold milk or eating something. The typical pain-food-relief is characteristic of the gastric ulcer whereas in duodenal ulcer, a patient experiences pain approximately 11/2 hrs after taking food.

Hurry, worry and curry are the root cause of most ulcers.
The common causes of ulcers are mainly:

- Irregular eating habits.
- Eating too much of spicy food.
- Drinking too much hot coffee, tea, alcohol and excessive smoking, chewing tobacco etc.
- Stress, strain and anxiety.
- Taking pain killers, anti-inflammatory drugs and steroids.
- Secretion of excess acid and loss of resistance of the inner mucosal lining of the stomach. Ulcers generally heal in about 3-4 weeks' time, but precautions taken later are important as they prevent recurrence.

Dietary guidelines:

- No solids should be consumed during active ulceration period. Only chilled milk, fully ripened banana, sapota, custard apple, apple stew should be given at an interval of every 2 hours.
- Fried and spicy non-vegetarian food irritates the mucus membrane and should be strictly avoided.
- Hot liquids like tea, coffee should be strictly avoided.

- Alcohol and smoking should be avoided.
- All citrus fruits and their juices should be strictly avoided.
- Avoid all fibrous foods as they cause mechanical irritation to the ulcer.
- Total physical and mental rest is very essential to lessen the vigorous contractions of stomach and to hasten the healing of ulcer.
- Once the condition improves, vegetable puree, non-spicy vegetable soups, custard and puddings can be included along with the milk diet.
- After a period of 4-6 weeks, bland, non-spicy, high protein and high carbohydrate diet is to be substituted gradually with normal food with adequate time gap between each meal.
- Too sweet and sour foods should be avoided.
- All refined flours, cornflours, pastries, cakes, jams and jellys should be avoided.
- Vegetable dalia, chapati and rice are good substitutes to cereal foods.
- Raw vegetables, sprouts and leafy vegetables should be avoided.
- Bananas, apples, custard apple, sapota, papaya can be taken.
- Pineapple, orange, guava, tomato should be avoided.
- Taking of small meals at regular intervals should be strictly adhered to.

Duodenitis

The innermost soft mucosal lining of the duodenum inflames in duodenitis resulting in problems similar to that of gastritis, except for the pain felt slightly above and right to the navel. Dietary guidelines are similar to the ones mentioned for gastritis.

Colitis

Colitis is inflammation of the large intestine or colon. It is generally of two types, mucus and ulcerative colitis.

Dietary guidelines:

- Initially fasting for a couple of days with buttermilk is advisable.
- Later, fruits like well ripened banana, papaya, custard apple, sapota should be given.
- Soothing diet, totally bland, soft cooked vegetables, rice or dalia should be continued at least for 3-6 months.
- Plenty of tender coconut water should be given.
- Cooked apple (stew) also helps in healing ulcers in the colon.
- Spices, condiments, tea, coffee, alcohol and smoking are to be avoided completely.
- Raw salads and leafy vegetables should be avoided as they contain high fibre.
- Food prepared out of refined flours, fried foods, pastries, cakes etc. should be avoided.

Diarrhoea

Frequent passage of loose stools is otherwise known as diarrhoea.

Causes:

1. Failure of water absorption capacity from the undigested wastes, due to mucosal disease, such as mucus colitis ulcerative colitis, amoebiasis etc.
2. Insufficient secretion of lactose enzyme leading to difficulty in digestion of milk.
3. Presence of inabsorbable substance in the tract formed by toxins, fatty acids etc.
4. Anxiety, fear, unaccustomed settings. However, diarrhoea is a natural phenomenon induced by fasting as self-healing force of the body to expel the toxins from the system rapidly.

The following simple remedies are good enough to control all forms of diarrhoea. However, after adopting some if one gets no relief, one should immediately seek the advice of an expert.

Dietary guidelines:

- Fast on buttermilk, curd or whey water to start with, for a couple of days.

- Later on, for a few days, one should remain on any of the items mentioned below:
  - (a) Well ripened banana, sapota, custard apple and naturally sweet curds.
  - (b) Sago kheer and banana.
  - (c) Curd rice and banana till loose motions come under control.
- Once the symptoms subside one should return to normal diet in a phased manner.
- Avoid cooked vegetables, raw salads, fruits such as orange mosambi, papaya, pineapple, apple etc. till the symptoms last.
- Avoid spices, sour things, citrus fruit juices etc.
- Drinking plenty of water is to be practised.

Constipation

It is a disease of modern civilisation and root cause of most of the other diseases.

Constipation depends upon number of factors such as area of distension of large bowel, rate and amount of pressure being exerted and the integrity of the nerves supplying to the large bowel area.

There are a number of causes for the constipation. They could be explained briefly as follows:

- ★ Faulty food intake, which includes irregular meal timings, eating junk, greasy, non-vegetarian foods made out of refined flours, and soft, non-bulk forming foods.
- ★ Lack of fibre in the food.
- ★ Lack of physical activity that causes the mobility of the colon, and using western type toilets to pass stools.
- ★ Failing to form a habit of early morning evacuation.
- ★ Failing to take sufficient fluids
- ★ Psychological aspects such as anxiety, worry, fear, unaccustomed setting and obsession with bowel evacuation habits
- ★ Number of diseases involving stomach, small and large intestines produce constipation
- ★ Medication adopted to control other diseases.

Dietary guidelines:

a) Generous use of fruits and raw vegetables such as carrot, radish lettuce, spinach, cauliflower, alfalfa, cabbage etc.

b) Use of whole wheat, wheat flour food preparations such as, brown bread, chapatis etc.

c) Use plenty of fibrous foods such as beans, bran, leafy vegetables, agar-agar, oatflakes, China grass, isabgol etc.

d) Generous intake of liquids such as water, lemon juice, fruit juices etc.

e) Use of confectioneries, pastries, cakes, sweets etc. should be curtailed.

f) All dry fruits, figs, prunes, raisins, apricots and plums, have laxative effect. And fresh fruits such as grapes, figs, papaya, banana, mango, grape fruit and orange are good and their use should he encouraged.

g) Taking 12 glasses of cold water immediately after getting up from bed and a casual stroll after that stimulates bowel movement.

h) Soaking dry fruits such as figs, raisins, dates or prunes in milk or plain water and taking it before going to bed or early in the morning is very useful in the treatment of constipation.

i) Mixing 2-3 tsp of isabgol in milk or warm water and taking it either at bedtime or early in the morning is also useful.

j) Sitting in squatting position for defaecation puts pressure on die lower abdomen which stimulates the bowel movement and hence use of Indian type toilet is beneficial.

Chronic amoebiasis

Vague abdominal discomfort, nausea, flatulence, pain in abdomen, occasionally loose motions with or without mucus and a feeling of illhealth are all characteristic features of chronic amoebiasis.

A majority of the people living in tropics are afflicted with this disease

Diet plays a very important role in controlling the growth and multiplication of the causative organism, entamoeba histolytica.

Dietary guidelines:

★ Fasting on buttermilk for 2-3 days or depending more on the endurance and individual capacity of the patient under the supervision of an expert.

★ After the fast, softer fruits such as banana, papaya, custard apple and sapota can be used.

★ A diet with curd rice and well ripened banana, both for lunch and dinner, is an excellent measure to reverse the condition.

★ All other guidelines given for constipation hold good for this also.

Obesity

Obesity and overweight complaints are quite common now. It, in fact, is a disease which leads to other fatal diseases such as diabetes, hypertension and heart attacks.

Though there are several causes for obesity, majority of the cases are due to overeating and lack of exercise.

Body weight is the simple index of fat. The logical way of losing weight is to cutdown food intake by 100 per cent without affecting the nutritive value of the food consumed and exercise regularly to burn the extra fat.

It is almost impossible to reduce extra fat by exercise alone. Exercise helps in burning fat by using the energy, but it is limited in scope. By a combination of sensible diet and regular exercise one can reduce weight reasonably better than by exercise alone.

Long term maintenance of weight

One kilogram of body fat contains roughly 7500 kcal energy. Suppose your requirement is roughly around 180 kcal/day, then if you reduce 250 kcal from regular food intake and burn another 250 kcal by exercise, total calorie reduction amounts to 500 kcal or roughly 3500 kcal per week, which is almost equal to 1/2 kg of body fat. By knocking out 250 kcals from diet and burning 250 kcals (walking at 8 kms/hr pace, 5 km/day, yogasanas for 1/2 hour and free hand exercises or sport for 1/2 hour) you lose at least 2 kgs/month, which is considered to be the safest method of losing weight.

Some people after losing weight fail to stick to the programme and probably due to lack of motivation and enthusiasm, tend to give up exercises, start eating more and gain weight. Temporary setbacks should not bother one. Here below are a few points, which weight watchers should always keep in mind for losing the weight till the desirable weight is reached and to maintain thereafter.

★ Do not overact either by cutting down too much or eating more, both are not advisable.

★ Do not expect a miracle. Some people take up dieting with an ambition and a target such as to get married, to get promotion, to look start etc. This is unrealistic thinking. Weight loss may solve the problems, but drastic measures are not advisable and they may lead to complications. Instead, one should forget one's desirable weight and start losing it gradually and in a long run.

Tips for reducing weight:

❖ Fast for longer periods say roughly upto 10-12 days under the supervision of experts at an institutional set up.

❖ Reduce butter, margarine, cooking fat (vanaspati), oil and fried food.

❖ Avoid:
   ◆ Cheese, cream and sweets.
   ◆ All non-vegetarian items.
   ◆ Rich sambar and soups. Pastries, biscuits, cakes and salted nuts. Sugary foods - jams, jellys, marmalades, sweets etc.
   ◆ Eating out and parties, especially late night parties.

❖ Stop alcohol, for alcohol is like fat. While 1 gm of fat yields 9 k calories, 1 gm of alcohol yields 7 k calories.

❖ Do not eat without knowing the calorific value of the food.

❖ Use only non-fat milk. (skimmed)

❖ Eat more watery vegetables such as all gourds and fruits, for they not only provide roughage but also minerals and vitamins and subsides the appetite. Above all they are low in calories.

❖ Eat fruit in between in case of hunger, but not along with the food.

Sample menu:

6.00 am	A glass of lime juice with honey
8.00 am	A fruit or buttermilk
12.00 am	100 gms raw salad, 300 gms vegetables,
to	3 chapatis/200 gms of rice/dalia/khichadi,
1 .00 pm	dal alternate days and buttermilk/soup
4.00 pm	Fruit juice / a juicy fruit
7.00 pm	2 or 3 varieties of fruits, each 100 gms, 200 gms steamed vegetables, and 1 tablespoon full of sprouts and soup.

Step by step eliminate all those things which tend to make you put on weight. For example, if you have eliminated fried food items wait till the craving for fried food is overcome and then shun the other item such as an ice-cream etc., making one change at a time.

❖ Keep a diary of your activity and your food intake. You will know for yourself where the mistake is.

❖ Eat slowly, avoid eating while reading or watching T.V., diversion while eating may lead to overeating. Eat the salad first and the rest of the food later on, chewing them properly. Do not drink water in between meals. Drink water half-an-hour before and one hour after the meal.

❖ Whenever you attend social gatherings or parties or eat out, speak up and do not feel shy to admit that you are dieting.

❖ Note your progress: Draw a graph with your initial weight as base to show your progress. Check your weight once in 3 days and record. Drawing a graph gives you immense pleasure and enthusiasm when once you start accomplishing the target aimed at

❖ If you lapse during dieting period, do not be disheartened. Temporary setbacks and lapses should not dampen your enthusiasm.

❖ Try, try again but do not lose heart. Maintenance of weight has to be done throughout the life. Temporary failures should not hamper the programme.

❖ Picture yourself as slim and visualise it everyday after yoganidra, for a better result.

Diseases of the Nervous System

Migraine and other forms of headaches

Headaches are of various types and are caused due to a variety of reasons such as tension, toxemia, congestion in blood, anaemia, sinusitis and wrong postures. Migraine is a type of headache which manifests with one side pain, associated by nausea, vomiting, blurring of vision, and intensifies with high frequency sounds and intense light. The episode lasts for a day or some times more.

The headache is caused by constipation. The undigested food remaining in the system purifies and produces toxins, which circulates in the blood stream causing headache. Migraine headache sets in as the toxin level in the blood reaches the saturation point.

Dietary guidelines:

- ✧ A short fast, to start with, to cleanse the blood stream.
- ✧ As constipation or indigestion is often the root cause of headaches, it has to be treated first.
- ✧ One should avoid eating tinned, stale, fried non-vegetable foods, sweets and spices.
- ✧ Irregular meal habits, late night heavy dinners should be avoided.

- A diet with 70 per cent fruits, vegetables, sprouts and 30 per cent cereals should be used.
- Avoid wrong combination of foods such as combination of starch, proteins and fatty foods.
- Eating between meals and drinking liquids should be avoided.
- Avoid drinking coffee, tea, cocoa, chocolate. smoking and alcohol.

Insomnia

On an average we require about 6-8 hours of sleep, when we do not get it we are said to be suffering from insomnia. Most common disorder of sleep is insomnia. Generally there are three types of insomnia:

- Difficulty in falling asleep.
- Awakening in the middle of night.
- Early morning awakening.

   Our health depends on how well we sleep. Not only the length of the sleep, even the depth and quality of the sleep is very important.

Dietary management for good sleep:

- A well balanced meal at properly regulated timings.
- Dine lightly to avoid digestive disturbances.
- Avoid drinking coffee, tea, cocoa, chocolate, alcohol and also smoking before going to bed to avoid gastritis.
- Avoid taking excess of liquids during night, for it may awaken you for urination, disturbing the sleep.
- In case of any difficulty in sleeping, drinking a glass of warm milk with honey/jaggery or hot honey water may help in getting sleep.

Menstrual Disorders

In the present set-up with the kind of lifestyle individuals lead, especially in the urban areas, 50 to 60 per cent of the menstruating women suffer from one type of menstrual problem or the other such as pre-menstrual tension, dysmenorrhea, polymenorrhea, scanty menstruation, lecorrhea, dysfunctional uterine, bleeding and problems at the time of menopause.

Several factors like defects in the genital organs (mechanical), hormonal, neurological and psychological play a role in the menstrual problems.

Dietary measures to be followed:

✧ Fasting 2-3 days during menstruation phase is advisable to provide physical, mental and psychological rest

✧ A well balanced food with restriction on salt, is essential as water retention before, during and after menstruation is quite common.

✧ Drink plenty of tender coconut water, barley water, dhania water or buttermilk as they have a diuretic effect.

✧ Drinking a glass of warm water with honey or warm milk with honey before going to bed relieves, fatigue and induces sleep. Efforts are to be made to maintain desirable weight.

The Urinary System

Kidneys are very important in maintenance of general health and elimination of waste. The accumulated wastes not eliminated by other excretory organs enter the blood stream and are filtered by the kidneys and eliminated as urea, uric acids, salts etc.

Diet plays a very important role in maintaining the health of the kidneys. If the food we take is of a good quality, the quality of blood flouting in the arteries will also be superior. Hence there will not be much burden on the kidneys.

A diet where meat, fish, eggs, cheese, starch, sugars and fat are predominant, causes strain on the kidneys, resulting in a high incidence of kidney disorders. Common disorders of the urino genital organs are, urinary tract infection, inflammation of the kidney, prostate gland enlargement (among aged) etc.

Another common urinary problem one suffers from is kidney or ureter stones obstructing the urinary flow. Stone generally comprises of calcium, uric acid or oxalic acid.

Dietary measures to be followed:
✧ Stop completely non-vegetarian food.
✧ Avoid all food items made out of refined flour, ghee, vanaspati.
✧ Avoid deep fried foods.
✧ Fasting 2-3 days on liquids is advantageous.
✧ Drink plenty of water to maintain normal urinary output.
✧ Drinking 2 glasses of water before going to bed in case of people with tendency to renal stone is advantageous.

✧ Use of plenty of tender coconut water, whey water, barley water, dhania water or buttermilk is very useful since they act like a diuretic.

✧ Foods containing purine (resulting in uric acid crystals), oxalic acid and calcium should be restricted by people who have tendency for formation of kidney stone. For foods, which contain high levels of purine oxalic acid and uric acid, may be referred to the tables given at the end of the book.

Allergy

Sensitivity to certain substances, which causes body reaction is known as allergy. General body reactions include; asthma, rhinitis, eczema, rashes, migraine, headaches and digestive disturbances.

The main cause of allergy is the food we consume. The food we eat may be well balanced, nutritious and good for some people, but the same time may be poisonous for others. Monitoring of food intake is very essential to find out what food item results in allergic manifestations, and for avoiding or substituting them with other food items. Balancing the diet, without depriving the body of the nutrition required, by avoiding foods to which one is allergic to is not an easy task, but is essential for one to remain healthy.

Allergy to certain food is quite common. Skin rashes and atopic eczema are due to milk and milk products, fish, pulses such as blackgram dal and bengalgram dal. Milk, soft drinks, tomatoes, oranges etc. may cause wheezing and rhinitis. Digestive disturbances are caused by milk and at times by gluten(protein) present in wheat. Preserved foods, sauces, food additives also cause allergy.

Milk is another controversial item, which causes allergy. In fact, after certain age milk is not recommended for several reasons. Soya milk would be an excellent substitute for cow's or buffalo's milk.

Some people are allergic to wheat, more to yeast, a substance used in making bread and gluten, a type of protein present in wheat, which results in chronic diseases such as ulcerative and mucus colitis. The earliest indication of allergy to wheat is when it causes indigestion or loose motion.

Method of food preparation also plays a very important role in checking allergic reactions. For example, soya should be soaked and the water discarded before being cooked. Most foods are less allergic, if cooked.

Dietary guidelines to be followed:

* Fast for 3-4 days to 1 week and then gradually come back to normal food in a phased manner.
* Record daily the food taken and the reaction if any, that follows.
* Do not eat between meals.
* Eat bland and fresh food with restriction on salt.
* Stop smoking and drinking alcohol.
* Avoid flavourings, odourants and additives
* Avoid processed, preserved and canned foods.
* Avoid foods made out of refined flour and deep fried.
* Avoid non-vegetarian food.
* Avoid coffee, tea, chocolate and instant drinks.
* Avoid honey, sugar, syrups etc.
* Once the condition improves and resistance developes, start eating potatoes, citrus fruits, nuts, cottage cheese, curds etc., and substitute milk with soya milk gradually.
* Change one at a time and if there is no reaction, continue the diet and if reaction persists stop it for another 2-3 days, go on bland diet and then include other items.
* It is good to stop taking non-vegetarian food, milk, cheese, white bread, cakes, pastries etc, for it is well known that they result in one or the other allergic reactions.
* To gain tolerance to the allowable food we eat, it is advisable to rotate them than taking the same diet always.

Acute diseases

All acute conditions such as fever, diarrhoea, rashes, cold, running nose etc., are nothing but direct manifestation of the self-healing power of the body. It subsides on its own after getting rid of the toxins built in the system.

Norman Consime author of the alltime best selling book of "Anatomy of illness'' says "Never underestimate the capacity of the human mind and body to regenerate even when the prospects seen are most wretched. The life force may be the least understood force on earth."

Fever

Raised body temperature often is the first indication that something is wrong with the system. Most of us act out of fear too early and treat the disease with antibiotics suppressing the bacterial activity for the time being. But if the same kind of negative lifestyle is continued we are sure to get another bout of fever. The frequent suppression of it with antibiotics leads to suppression of the immune response itself to the micro-organisms.

Fever is left best to run its course and that is the best remedy one could think of. Once the temperature comes down, one feels more energetic.

Dietary guidelines:

* Fast 2-3 days or extend further till the symptoms persist under the supervision of a naturopath.
* Drink plenty of water so that toxins are flushed out through urine and sweat.
* After breaking the fast, gradually start taking fruits. Eat plenty of citrus fruits, for they contain fair amount of vitamin C, which helps in building up resistance.
* Later switch over to cereals in the ideal combination of 70 per cent alkaline forming foods, such as fruit and vegetable and 30 per cent acid forming foods such as cereals.

All ordinary fevers should be treated in the above way. But some treatments for symptomatic relief could be given (Refer to Nature Cure Treatment book of INYS publications).

Seek the assistance of doctor if the fever does not subside even after a week and after the simple remedial measures have been taken.

Miracles of Water Therapy

Several chronic diseases for which no cure has been found, can be cured by a simple method called water therapy. The Japanese Sickness Association confirms that several diseases such as headache, hypertension, obesity, diabetes, arthritis, rheumatism, sinusitis, rhinitis, bronchitis, bronchial asthma, hyperacidity, gastritis, dysentery, constipation, irregular menstruation, urogenital problems etc., are cured by water therapy.

Though it sounds incredible, it has been proved factual and is recommended by several doctors as well. Human health depends mainly on the digestive system. As Swamy Paramahamesa Yogananda said, it is overeating all the 365 days of a year, that leads to most of the diseases.

Drinking ordinary potable water helps clean the gastrointestinal tract and the blood, thereby removes toxins from the body. Thus many of the ailments are cured by practising water therapy.

How to practise?

The method of water therapy is simple, easy and inexpensive. Early in the morning, before attending to any of the morning chores, 5 glasses of water (1.26 kg. or 12.60 cc) should be taken at one stretch. You may give a short break. Do spot walking exercise for a few minutes and then drink the rest of water. Take necessary precaution against impurities of water. Water should be boiled and cooled if purity is suspected.

For the next 45 minutes to one hour after drinking water, no other beverage or eatable should be taken. After supper one should not have any stimulating beverage or a soft drink.

During the first few days of therapy, one may pass urine 3-4 times within one hour after drinking water. Some may have even loose stools. But in a short period everything comes back to normalcy and symptoms of relief from the disease will be seen.

Persons suffering from arthritis and rheumatism should take Water Therapy three times a day in the first week and thereafter may practise it once a day. While practising Water Therapy, water should be taken two hours after each meal and not before that.

A boy who followed this therapy sums up his experience thus, "After drinking water, I urinated three times in one hour. Later breakfast tasted wonderful. The next day my bowels were free. In three months I put on weight. Ever since I took to Water Therapy, I never fell sick nor was I affected by cold or cough."

Experiments show that the following diseases can be cured by Water Therapy within the periods mentioned in the brackets.

Hypertension (one month), diabetes (one to two weeks), gastritis (one week) and constipation (one or two days).

PART III

RECIPES

Soups

TOMATO SOUP

Calories -180   *Serves -4*

Ingredients

Tomato – ½ kg
Bottlegourd – 250 gm
Coriander power – 1 tsp
Ginger – 2 tsp
Jaggery – 10 gms
Asafoetida – a pinch

Salt – to taste
Curry leaves, cumin seeds,
celery leaves and coriander
leaves a little.
Oil – ½ tsp
Water – 800 ml

METHOD

1. Boil tomato, bottlegourd, salt and coriander powder in 800 ml water.
2. When cooked, strain and keep the water aside. Blend the boiled vegetables in a mixie and extract the juice. Add jaggery to the water.
3. Mix this puree with the water kept aside. Season it with oil, cumin seeds, asafoetida, celery leaves and curry leaves.
4. Garnish with coriander leaves.

GREEN PEAS SOUP

Calories -150   *Serves -3*

Ingredients

Peas – 100 gm   Lemon – 1
Milk – 100 ml   Salt – to taste
                                   Water – 500 ml

METHOD

1. Boil green peas till it becomes soft. Drain water and keep it aside (500 ml water)
2. Blend the peas into a paste. Add drained water and milk.
3. Boil the mixture for 5 minutes by adding salt to taste.
4. Serve hot with coriander leaves and lemon juice.

VARIATION

1. Dried peas can be used in place of fresh peas.
2. Substitute coconut milk for milk. Also add half a cup of carrot juice.

CREAM OF CARROT SOUP

Calories -338   *Serves -4*

Ingredients

Carrot – 250 gms   Milk – 100 ml
Potato – 75 gms   Salt and pepper – to taste
Fresh cream – 30 gms   Water – 1 lit

METHOD

1. Chop vegetables. Add six tea cups of water and cook in a pressure cooker.
2. Blend the mixture in a liquidiser and strain.
3. Boil for 15 minutes, add cream, milk, salt and pepper. Serve hot.

Note: When serving for the patients undergoing naturopathy treatments, avoid fresh cream and use skimmed milk.

VARIATION

Substitute carrot with tomatoes. Those who like onions and potatoes may add one or two of either to enhance the flavour and taste.

SNAKE GOURD SOUP

Calories -377   *Serves -6*

Ingredients

Snake gourd – 1 kg   Water – 1.5 ltrs
Moong dal – 30 gms   Cumin seeds – ½ tsp
Potato – 50 gms   Salt and lime juice – to taste
Oil – 1 tsp   Parsley/Coriander leaves – a few

METHOD

1. Chop snake gourd and potatoes.
2. Fry moong dal and cumin seeds in oil till a roasted aroma emanates.
3. Add this to the vegetables along with 2-3 cups of water. Steam for ten minutes.
4. When cool, mash and grind. Strain through a coarse sieve. Boil for 5 minutes.
5. Add salt and lime juice and garnish with coriander leaves.

Note: For persons not undergoing treatment, half a spoon of powdered black pepper and a cup of milk added to the soup will enhance its taste.

VARIATIONS

a. ½ kg palak/spinach and ½ kg bottle gourd.
b. ½ kg pumpkin and ½ kg bottle gourd.
c. ½ kg cabbage and two vegetable marrows (Chow-Chow).
d. ½ kg cabbage, ½ kg spinach and ¼ kg bottle gourd.
e. ½ kg carrot, ½ kg cabbage and 3-4 tomatoes.
f. 1 kg ridge gourd and one potato.

ASHGOURD SOUP

Calories -123   **Serves -4**

Ingredients

Ashgourd – 450 gms   Salt – to taste
Onion – 50 gms (optional)   Coriander leaves – a few
Potatoes – 50 gms   Water – 800 ml
Tomato – 25 gms

METHOD

1. Chop the vegetables. Add seven cups of water and steam them in a pressure cooker.
2. Mash well and filter. Add salt.
3. Boil for 5 minutes and garnish with coriander leaves.

MIXED VEGETABLES SOUP

Calories -1235   **Serves -4**

Ingredients

Tomato – 100 gms   Spinach – 100 gms
Cucumber – 100 gms   Peas – 50 gms
Beetroot – 100 gms   Salt – to taste
Cabbage – 100 gms   Water – 800 ml

METHOD

1. Chop the vegetables and steam them in a pressure cooker.
2. Separate the liquid and vegetables. Blend vegetables into a creamy pulp. Sieve it.
3. Mix with the liquid kept aside. Add salt. Boil for 5 minutes.
4. Season with oil and cumin seeds. Serve with a piece of lemon.

Note: Any other seasonal vegetable may be added. Coconut gratings and green coriander leaves may be used for garnishing.

CUCUMBER SOUP

Calories -210   *Serves -4*

Ingredients

Cucumber – 1 kg   Salt – to taste
Onion – 50 gms   Pepper – to taste
Oil – 1 tsp   Water – 800 ml
Mushroom – 25 gms

METHOD

1. Peel a cucumber and boil it in four cups of water, liquidise and sieve.
2. Cut onion and mushroom into small pieces.
3. Heat oil, fry onion to golden brown. Fry mushrooms lightly in the same oil.
4. Add to cucumber stock and boil. Serve with salt and pepper.

VARIATION

Vegetable stock can be used to improve the taste.

FRENCH ONION SOUP

Calories -135   *Serves -3*

Ingredients

Rice – 20 gms   Oil – ½ tsp
Carrot – 15 gms   Salt, pepper, lime and coriander
Tomato – 50 gms   leaves – to taste
Onion – 50 gms   Water – 500 ml

METHOD

1. Chop onion finely and fry in oil to golden brown, keep aside.
2. Cook rice, carrot and tomato in two cups of water, liquidise and strain.
3. Mix onion to strained juice, add salt, pepper and boil.
4. Serve with lime juice and coriander leaves.

RAJMA SOUP

Calories -90   *Serves -2*

Ingredients

Rajma – 25 gms (soaked)   Coriander leaves – to taste
Carrot – 10 gms   Water – 400 ml
Salt, red chilli , lime,

METHOD

1. Cook rajma and carrot in two cups of water, liquidise and strain.
2. Boil the strained water with salt and chilli powder.
3. Serve with lime and coriander leaves.

POTATO BASED TURDAL SOUP

Calories -86   *Serves -2*

Ingredients

Potato – 10 gms   Water – 400 ml
Turdal – 15 gms   Seasoning oil – ½ tsp
Coriander leaves, salt, green   Mustard – ½ tsp
chilli, lime – to taste

METHOD
Same as other soups.

VARIATION
Cabbage + beetroot + potato

PAPAYA SOUP

Calories -47   *Serves -2*

Ingredients

Raw/half ripe papaya – 100 gms   *Lime, salt, coriander, pepper – as required*
Carrot – 2 gms   *Water – 400 ml*

METHOD
Same as other soups.

TOMATO, CUCUMBER AND CAPSICUM SOUP

Calories -93   *Serves -2*

Ingredients

Tomato – 250 gms   *Onion – 20 gms*
Capsicum – 25 gms   *Salt + pepper + lime + coriander-to taste*
Cucumber – 200 gms   *Water – 300 ml*

METHOD
Same as other soups.

CUCUMBER AND MINT SOUP

Calories -96   *Serves -3*

Ingredients

Cucumber   100 gms   *Salt, pepper, lime – to taste*
Mint – 15 gms   *Rice – 20 gms*
Onion – 15 gms   *Water – 500 ml*

METHOD
Same as other soups.

PEAS MUSHROOM SOUP

Calories -228   *Serves -5*

Ingredients

Green peas – 25 gms   Paneer – 10 gms
Mushrooms – 15 gms   Salt, pepper and lime – to taste
Milk – 200 ml   Water – 600 ml
Bread crumbs – 10 gms

METHOD

1. Cook green peas and mushrooms in just enough water till they become soft.
2. Liquidise and strain. Add milk, bread crumbs and grated paneer. Bring to a boil.
3. Add salt, pepper and serve with lime.

VARIATIONS

Use oats in place of green peas – 25 gms. Fry mushrooms in a little ghee and add to oats gruel.

CAPSICUM SOUP

Calories -75   *Serves -2*

Ingredients

Tomato – 100 gms   Oil – ½ tsp
Capsicum – 100 gms   Salt – to taste
Garlic – 4 cloves   Water – 800 ml
Clove – 1

METHOD

1. Boil tomato and garlic. When it is soft, liquidise and strain.
2. Cut capsicum into small pieces. Fry in oil for 5 minutes and add it to the soup.
3. Add salt and serve.

VEGETABLE LAPSI SOUP

Calories -215   **Serves -4**

Ingredients

Cabbage – 250 gms   *Dalia – 1tbsp*
Cucumber – 150 gms   *Salt, pepper and lime – to taste*
Green peas – 50 gms   *Water – 800 ml*

METHOD
1. Chop all the ingredients and cook in a pressure cooker in sufficient water. Liquidise and strain.
2. Add salt and pepper. Boil and serve with lime.
3. Garnish with coriander leaves.

APPLE OATS SOUP

Calories -225   **Serves -5**

Ingredients

Apple – 150 gms   *Salt/Jaggery – to taste*
Oats – 10 gms   *Water – 1 lit*
Milk – 150 ml

METHOD
1. Peel and cut apple. Mix with oats and boil in water. Cool, liquidise and strain.
2. Add milk, salt/jaggery. Heat before serving.
3. Garnish with a few pieces of apple.

FENUGREEK METHI SOUP

Calories -104   *Serves -3*

Ingredients

Fenugreek leaves – 200 gms   Jeera powder – ½ tsp
Tomato – 30 gms   Salt – to taste
Dhaniya powder – ½ tsp.   Water – 700 ml

METHOD

1. Pressure cook fenugreek leaves and tomato, liquidise and strain.
2. Add the remaining ingredients and boil. Serve hot.

CAULIFLOWER SOUP

Calories -380   *Serves -6*

Ingredients

Cauliflower – 300 gms   Wheat flour – 2 tbsp
Onion – 100 gms   Milk – 200 ml
Ginger – 2" piece   Salt, lime and pepper – to taste
Green chilli – 1   Oil – ½ tsp
                                                    Water – 1 1/2 lit

METHOD

1. Chop onion and cauliflower and fry in oil for 2-3 minutes.
2. Add wheat flour and fry for one more minute. Add green chilli, ginger and pressure cook.
3. Cool, liquidise and strain it. Reheat, add salt and milk. Serve with lime and pepper powder.

Salad

ONION TOMATO

Calories -108   *Serves -3*

Ingredients

Onion – 25 gms   Cucumber – 100 gms
Tomato – 10 gms   Cabbage leaves – 50 gms
Carrot – 100 gms   Chopped mint – ½ tsp
                                  Pepper – ¼ tsp

METHOD
Cut all the ingredients and mix with salt, lime and pepper.

TOMATO ALFALFA

Calories -17   *Serves -1*

Ingredients

Cucumber – 50 gms   Sprouted alfalfa – 5 gms
Tomato – 10 gms   Grated carrot – 1 tsp
Capsicum – 10 gms

METHOD
Slice cucumber and tomato and arrange in a salad bowl. Place sprouted alfalfa at the centre and garnish with carrot.

APPLE CANAPES

Calories -650   *Serves -5*

Ingredients

Apple – 300 gms (2-3)
Cottage cheese – 125 gms (1/2 cup)
Celery – 50 gms (3 tbsp chopped)

Onion – 25 gms (1 or 2 small)
Curry powder – 1 tsp
Salt – to taste

METHOD

1. Chop onion and washed cerely leaves.
2. Core and slice the apples. Mix cheese and seasoning (onion, curry powder, celery and salt). Spread on the apple slices.

VARIATION

Omit seasoning and use a bit of cheese between two slices of apple. Recommended for people who have good digestion and appetite. However for patients, less cheese should be used.

RECHTER SALAD

Calories -238   *Serves -7*

Ingredients

Carrot (grated) – 550 gms
Beetroot (grated) – 50 gms
Turnip (grated) – 15 gms
Radish (grated) – 30 gms
Parsley (chopped) – 15 gms
Tomato (sliced) – 50 gms
Palak (chopped) – 15 gms
Ajwain leaves (chopped) – gms
Cabbage leaves (chopped) – 20 gms

Cucumber (sliced) – 50 gms
Prepare masala from the following
Til – 1 tbsp
Coriander powder – 1/2 tsp
Cumin powder – 1/2 tsp
Sunflower oil – 5 drops
Lemon juice – 5 drops
Salt – to taste

METHOD

1. Add masala to the sliced cucumber and tomato, mix well, transfer cucumber and tomato to a salad bowl.
2. Dress with grated carrot, beetroot, turnip, radish chopped parsley, lettuce, cabbage, ajwain leaves and palak.
3. Roast a little til, make a coarse powder and sprinkle before sewing.
4. Melon and pumpkin seeds may also be used in the same manner.

MIXED VEGETABLE SALAD

Calories -115.0   *Serves -4*

Ingredients

Small lettuce – 25 gms	Lemon – 1
Radish – 250 gms	Gingelly oil – 1 tsp
Tomato – 100 gms	Garlic – 1 clove

METHOD

1. Chop all the vegetables into small pieces and mix together.
2. Dress with gingelly oil and crushed garlic.

SUMMER RETREAT

Calories -70   *Serves -2*

Ingredients

Cucumber – 100 gms	Lemon – 1
Tomato – 100 gms	Honey – 1 tbsp
Onion – 30 gms	Salt – to taste

METHOD

1. Slice cucumber, onion and tomato finely. Add half a tablespoon of honey and lemon juice.
2. Add salt to taste. Garnish with coriander or pudina leaves. This salad is most welcome in summer.

APPLE, CARROT AND RAISING SALAD

Calories -278.0   *Serves -2*

Ingredients

Apple – 100 gms	*Cream – 20 gms (optional)*
Raisins – 20 gms	*Salt – a pinch*
Carrot – 25 gms	*Lemon juice – 2 tbsp*

METHOD
1. Chop the apple, grated carrot, mix with raisins and salt.
2. Add cream and lemon juice.

MIXED FRUIT SALAD

Calories -3,600   *Serves -30*

Ingredients

Banana – 500 gms	*Apple – 200 gms*
Orange – 100 gms	*Pineapple – 250 gms*
Grapes – 100 gms	*Jaggery – 1/2 kg*
Papaya – 250 gms	*Milk – 1 lit*
Dates – 100 gms	*Cardamom powder – 3/4 tsp*

METHOD
1. Boil milk and cool. Mix jaggery in a little milk, boil and filter.
2. Cut all the fruits into small pieces and mix lightly with cold milk and jaggery.
3. Add a little cardamom powder. Keep in a refrigerator. Serve cold.

CARROT AND CHEESE SALAD

Calories -258   **Serves -6**

Ingredients

Carrot – 200 gms   Orange – 60 gms
Cheddar cheese – 30 gms   Dried fruit and nuts – 1 tbsp

METHOD
1. Peel and grate carrots. Chop orange.
2. Mix all the ingredients together and serve as a side dish/main meal.

Note: As an alternative, add apples, onions or tomatoes for a low fat diet.

CABBAGE KOSAMBRI

Calories -40   **Serves -1**

Ingredients

Cabbage – 50 gms   Coriander leaves – a few
Oil – 1/2 tsp   Salt and lemon juice – to taste
Mustard – 1/2 tsp

METHOD
1. Cut cabbage into small pieces. Add salt and lime juice.
2. Season with oil and mustard. Garnish with coriander leaves.

VARIATION
1. Roasted and powdered groundnut can be added or sprouted groundnut can be used.

GREEN SALAD

Calories -41   *Serves -1*

Ingredients

Methi leaves – 25 gms   Cucumber – 30 gms
Pineapple – 25 gms   Onion (optional)
Carrot – 25 gms   Lime juice and salt – to taste

METHOD
1. Chop all the vegetables and fruit. Mix with lime and salt.

VARIATION
Radish, apple, carrot (combination)

SPROUT SALAD

Calories -112   *Serves -3*

Ingredients

Moong sprouted – 25 gms   Coriander salt and lime – to
Cabbage – 25 gms   taste
Carrot – 50 gms

METHOD
1. Chop cabbage, grate carrot and mix with moong sprouts.
2. Add salt, lime juice and garnish with coriander leaves.

CALIFORNIA COLESLAW

Calories -161   *Serves -4*

Ingredients

Cabbage – 200 gms   Lime juice – 1 tsp
Apple – 100 gms   Salt and coriander leaves – to
Orange – 100 gms   taste

METHOD
1. Grate cabbage. Core apple and peel orange.
2. Mix the fruit mixture along with lime juice, salt and coriander leaves.

GREEN GRAM DAL SALAD

Calories -187   *Serves -3*

Ingredients

Green gram dal – 50 gms   Lime, salt, green chillies and
Cucumber – 100 gms   coriander leaves – to taste

METHOD
1. Pressure cook green gram dal with very little water. (Dal should not become mashy).
2. Chop cucumber, green chillies and coriander leaves. Add salt and lime juice to the dal.
3. Seasoning is optional.

TOMATO SALAD WITH FRENCH DRESSING

Calories -100   *Serves -3*

Ingredients

Tomato – 100 gms   Lemon juice – 1 tsp
Cucumber – 120 gms   Salt and mustard powder – to
Cauliflower – 100 gms   taste
French dressing corn oil – 1 tsp

METHOD
1. Mix the ingredients of French dressing in a mixie.
2. Cut all the vegetables and mix well with dressing.

VARIATION
Only in dressing:
1. Corn oil in equal quantity
2. Lemon juice as desired
3. Salt
4. Mustard powder, pepper powder and crushed garlic 2-3.

SPRING SALAD BOWL

Calories -160   *Serves -3*

Ingredients

Lettuce – 100 gms   Onion – 50 gms
Radish – 100 gms   Tomato – 50 gms
Cucumber – 200 gms   Salt – to taste
                            Honey – 10 ml

METHOD
1. Shred lettuce, cut tomatoes into small pieces.
2. Add chopped radish, diced cucumber and onions. Pour honey and salt and mix well. Serve immediately.

Combinations of salads:

1. Cucumber + chakramani + lime + salt + seasoning ingredients.
2. Pineapple + cucumber + tomato salad
3. Pineapple + carrot + capsicum salad
4. Onion + tomato + carrot + cucumber + cabbage leaves + mint + lime juice + salt + pepper.
5. Beetroot + curds + cucumber + salt + coriander leaves + seasoning.

Chutneys

CHANNAPUTANA CHUTNEY

Calories -600   *Serves -6*

Ingredients

Channaputana – 100 gms   Lime juice – 2 tsp
Coconut – 100 gms   Salt – to taste
Coriander leaves – 25 gms   Garlic and ginger (optional)
Green chillies – 1

METHOD

1. Except for lime juice, grind all the ingredients to a coarse paste. Then add the lime juice and mix well.
2. If required, seasoning may be done.

VARIATION

a. In place of channaputana, fried bengalgram dal can be used.
b. Only coconut can be used, omitting dals.

BRINJAL CHUTNEY

Calories -112   *Serves -3*

Ingredients

Round brinjal – 100 gms   *Salt, red chillies and lime –*
Coconut – 20 gms   *to taste.*

METHOD
Roast brinjal, remove the outer skin, grind along with other ingredients to a smooth paste.

VARIATION
1. Soaked bengalgram and finely chopped onion can be added.
2. Season the chutney.

GROUNDNUT CHUTNEY

Calories -141   *Serves -2*

Ingredients

Groundnut – 25 gms   *coriander leaves – to taste*
and chilli powder, salt, lime,   *Garlic and ginger (optional)*

METHOD
1. Grind all the ingredients to a fine paste.
2. Season (optional)

MINT CHUTNEY

Calories -48   *Serves -2*

Ingredients

Mint – 100 gms   *Lime/Mango (raw)/Tamarind*
Green chilli – 1   *and salt – to taste*
Ginger – a small piece

METHOD

1. Cut and grind all the ingredients together.
2. Season with oil and mustard seeds (optional).

VARIATION

In place of mint, coriander/curry leaves can be used.

APPLE CHUTNEY

Calories -96   *Serves -2*

Ingredients

Apple – 100 gms   Channaputana – 10 gms
Green chilli – 1   Salt and lime – to taste

METHOD

1. Remove the seeds of apple and cut into small pieces.
2. Grind along with other ingredients to a chutney consistency.
3. Season it with mustard, oil and jeera (optional)

MANGO CHUTNEY

Calories -148   *Serves -3*

Ingredients

Raw mango – 200 gms
Salt and jaggery – to taste
Green chilli – 1
Oil Mustard seeds (optional)

METHOD

1. Wash and chop the mango. Grind along with other ingredients to a chutney consistency.
2. Season with oil and mustard seeds (optional).

AMLA CHUTNEY

Calories -58   *Serves -2*

Ingredients

Amla – 100 gms   *(optional)*
Green chilli – 1   *Salt and jaggery – to taste.*
Ginger and garlic – a little   *Jeera and oil (optional)*

METHOD
1. Remove seeds from amla. Grind with other ingredients to a smooth paste.
2. Season with jeera and oil (optional)

CARROT CHUTNEY

Calories -48   *Serves -2*

Ingredients

Carrot – 100 gms   *Salt and lime – to taste*
Green chilli – 1   *Jaggery – to taste*
Ginger – a small piece

METHOD
1. Chop carrot, grind along with other ingredients to a smooth paste.
2. Season with oil and mustard.

ONION CHUTNEY

Calories -95   *Serves -2*

Ingredients

Onion – 100 gms   Salt, jaggery and lime – to taste
Red chilli – 1   Channaputana – 25 gms
Oil – 1 tsp

METHOD
1. Fry onion (chopped) and red chilli in oil and grind to a fine paste along with other ingredients.
2. Season with oil, mustard and curry leaves (optional).

TOMATO CHUTNEY

Calories -40   *Serves -2*

Ingredients

Tomato – 200 gms   Green chilli – 1
Ginger – small pieces   Tamarind and salt – to taste
Garlic – 2 cloves   Curry leaves – a few

METHOD
1. Roast the tomatoes.
2. Grind along with other ingredients to a thick paste.
3. Season with oil and mustard.

RAW PAPAYA CHUTNEY

Calories -185   *Serves -2*

Ingredients

Raw papaya – 500 gms   Lime, pepper powder and salt –
Roasted cumin seeds – 1/2 tsp   to taste
                                 Coriander leaves – a few

METHOD
1. Peel the skin of papaya and grate. Pressure cook and grind.
2. Mix with other ingredients.

RIDGE GOURD (TORI) CHUTNEY

Calories -106   *Serves -1*

Ingredients

Ridgegourd – 100 gms   Oil – 1/2 tsp
Coconut – 1 tbsp   Mustard – 1/2 tsp
Red chilli – 1   Lime, salt and jaggery – to taste

METHOD
Peel the skin and pressure cook the ridgegourd. Grind it with other
ingredients to a fine paste and season.

CHOW-CHOW MARROW CHUTNEY

Calories -93.6   *Serves -2*

Ingredients

Chow-chow marrow – 100 gms   Red chilli – 1
Coconut – 1 tbsp   Lime, salt and jaggery – to taste

METHOD
Remove the skin of chow-chow marrrow. Pressure cook and grind
along with other ingredients. Then season.

SESAME CHUTNEY

Calories -50   **Serves -2**

Ingredients

Sesame seeds – 100 gms   Cumin seeds – 1/2 tsp
Green chilli – 1   Coriander leaves – a few
Garlic – 2 cloves   Salt, jaggery and lime – to taste.

METHOD
1. Roast cumin and sesame seeds.
2. Grind along with other ingredients to a smooth paste.
3. Season with oil, mustard and curry leaves (optional).

APPLE STEW

Calories -68   **Serves -2**

Ingredients

Apple – 200 gm
Honey – 1 tsp

METHOD
1. Steam the apples, blend in a mixer till the pulp is homogenized.
2. Serve chilled with a teaspoonful of honey.

Recommended:

For patients suffering from hyperacidity, stomach ulcer and muscular cramps in the legs due to potassium and calcium deficiency. It is easy to digest and helps to relieve diarrhoea. It is good even for cancer patients.

MULI PACHADI

Calories -80   *Serves -2*

Ingredients

Tender radish leaves –   Salt and lime – to taste
100 gms   Turmeric powder – a pinch
Radish – 50 gms   Cumin seeds – 1/2 tsp
Oil – 1 tsp

METHOD

1. Shred radish leaves and cut radish finely. Season with oil, cumin seeds and turmeric powder.
2. Add salt and lime juice to taste. Serve with hot rotis.

Sprouts

GREEN GRAM SPROUTS

Calories -361   *Serves -3*

Ingredients

Moong sprouts – 100 gms   Coriander leaves – a few
Lettuce leaves – 20 gms   Salt – to taste
Lemon juice – 1/2 tsp   Coconut gratings – 1 tbsp

METHOD

Mix all the ingredients. Garnish with coconut gratings or carrot.

WHEAT SPROUTS

Calories -389   *Serves -5*

Ingredients

Wheat sprouts – 100 gms   Lemon and salt – to taste
Parsley – 50 gms (chopped)   Coconut gratings – 1 tbsp.

METHOD

Same as other sprouts salad.

TOMATO AND ALFALFA SPROUTS

Calories -90   *Serves -4*

Ingredients

Tomato – 50 gms   Lime and salt – to taste
Alfalfa – 150 gms   Coriander leaves – a few

METHOD
Same as other sprouts.

MOONG SPROUT SALAD

Calories -900   *Serves -12*

Ingredients

Moong sprouts – 25gms   Coriander leaves – a few
Chopped onion – 25 gms   Sesame oil – 1 tsp
Chopped tomatoes – 25 gms   Lemon and salt – to taste

METHOD
Same as other salads.

MIXED SPROUT SALAD

Calories -767   *Serves -8*

Ingredients

Wheat sprouts – 100 gms   Parsley chopped – 100 gms
Moong sprouts – 100 gms   Salt and lime – to taste
Alfalfa sprouts – 100 gms

METHOD
Same as other sprout salads.

Combinations:

1. Groundnut sprouts + beetroot grated + coriander leaves + lime + salt.
2. Wheat sprouts + beetroot grated + coriander leaves + lime + salt.
3. Moong sprouts + jaggery + coconut.
4. Moong sprouts + coconut + seasoning.
5. Groundnut + carrot (grated) + lime + salt.
6. Moong sprouts + carrot (grated) + lime + salt + coriander leaves.

Raitas

PINEAPPLE RAITA

Calories -410   *Serves -6*

Ingredients

Pineapple – 500 gms   Cardamom powder – 5 gms
Thick curds – 150 ml   Jaggery – 15 gms
Milk – 50 ml   Raisins and dates – a few

METHOD
1. Cut pineapple into small pieces and mix with other ingredients.
2. Garnish with raisins and dates. Serve cold.

BEETROOT RAITA

Calories -275   *Serves -4*

Ingredients

Beetroot – 200 gms   Oil – 1 tsp
Thick curds – 200 gms   Mustard – 1 tsp
Coconut scrapings – 1 tsp   Turmeric – a pinch
                              Coriander leaves – a few

METHOD
1. Same as other raitas. Season the raita with oil, mustard and turmeric.

TOMATO RAITA

Calories -80   **Serves -2**

Ingredients

Tomato – 100 gms   Coriander leaves – a few
Thick curds – 100 gms   Salt – to taste

METHOD
Same as other raitas. Season if desired.

BANANA RAITA

Calories -450   **Serves -5**

Ingredients

Ripened banana – 250 gms   Salt – to taste
Curds – 150 gms   Mustard and cumin powder – 1
Coconut gratings – 1 tbsp   tsp each

METHOD
Same as other raitas. Serve cold.

RAINBOW RAITA

Calories -194   **Serves -4**

Ingredients

Thick curds – 150 gms   Tamarind juice – 1 tbsp
Potatoes – 100 gms   Salt – to taste
Mint – 15 gms

METHOD
1. Boil potato and cut into cubes
2. Grind mint to a paste. Mix all the ingredients in beaten curds.

PAPAYA RAITA

Calories -86   **Serves -2**

Ingredients

Ripe papaya – 100 gms   Jaggery – 15 gms
Curds – 50 gms   Salt – to taste

METHOD
Same as other raitas.

CUCUMBER RAITA

Calories -185   **Serves -4**

Ingredients

Cucumber – 500 gms   Salt – to taste
Curds – 200 gms   Coriander leaves – a few

METHOD
Chop or grate cucumber. Follow the same method as other raitas.

POTATO ONION RAITA

Calories -175   **Serves -3**

Ingredients

Potato – 100 gms   Oil – half tsp
Onion – 25 gms   Mustard – half tsp
Curds – 50 gms   Coriander leaves – a few
Salt – to taste   Grated coconut – 1 tsp
                                          (optional)

METHOD
1. Steam potato, peel the skin and mash.
2. Chop onion and coriander leaves. Beat curds and mix all the ingredients.
3. Season with oil and mustard. Serve with chapati.

Cereal Preparations

CHINESE RICE

Calories -2391   *Serves -8*

Ingredients

Rice – 500 gms   Onion – 50 gms
Beans – 200 gms   Soya sauce – 5 tsp
Carrot – 200 gms   Oil – 10 gms
Peas – 150 gms   Celery stem – a few
                                  Salt – to taste

METHOD

1. Wash and cook rice in sufficient water. Cool the rice by spreading on a plate.
2. Half cook carrots, beans, peas, celery stem and onion with salt and little oil. Continue cooking for 2 to 3 minutes.
3. Mix soya sauce to rice and add the mixture to vegetables. Serve hot.

LEMON RICE

Calories -1140   *Serves -4*

Ingredients

Rice – 250 gms   *Urad dal – 1 tbsp*
Oil – 3 tbsp   *Lime juice – to taste*
Mustard – 1 tbsp   *Turmeric powder – a pinch*
Salt – to taste   *Curry and coriander leaves - a few*

METHOD

1. Cook rice in sufficient water. Cool the rice by spreading on a plate.
2. Heat oil, add mustard, dal and curry leaves. Fry till the dal is golden brown. Add turmeric powder.
3. Add seasoned mixture, lemon juice, salt and coriander leaves to rice and mix well.

VARIATION

Grated carrots/boiled peas can be added to it.

TURDAL KHICHADI

Calories -1470   *Serves -7*

Ingredients

Rice – 250 gms   *Turmeric powder – a pinch*
Turdal – 100 gms   *Cumin seeds – ½ tbsp*
Oil – 2 tbsp   *Curry leaves – a few*
Mustard – ½ tbsp   *Salt – to taste*

METHOD I

1. Soak rice and dal for half an hour separately.
2. Cook dal in sufficient water till half done. Then add rice and water. Continue cooking till rice is cooked.
3. Season with oil, cumin seeds, turmeric powder and curry leaves.
4. Add salt and mix thoroughly. Serve hot.

METHOD II
1. Season with oil, mustard, curry leaves and turmeric
2. Add soaked dal and rice. Put every thing in a pressure cooker. Pour 1:3 ratio (1 part of rice, 3 parts of water).
3. Add salt and mix well. Serve with kadi.

Note : This should not be given to asthma patients.

VEGETABLE KHICHADI

Calories -1114   *Serves -6*

Ingredients

Carrots – 100 gms	Oil – 15 gms
Beans – 100 gms	Cumin seeds – 1 tsp
Cabbage – 100 gms	Turmeric – a pinch
Peas – 50 gms	Salt – to taste
Green gram dal – 75 gms	Curry leaves – a few
Rice – 150 gms	

METHOD
1. Heat oil, add cumin seeds and curry leaves.
2. Wash and cut all the vegetables, then add to seasoned vessel.
3. Wash rice and moong dal. Pour all the ingredients into a pressure cooker. Add salt and water in 1:3 ratio - (for 1 part of rice 3 parts of water) and pressure cook.

CORIANDER RICE

Calories -600   *Serves -4*

Ingredients

Rice – 150 gms   Beans – 50 gms
Coriander leaves – 60 gms   Green chillies – 2
Garlic – 3-4 cloves   Oil – 15 gms
Carrot – 50 gms   Salt – to taste

METHOD

1. Make a paste of coriander leaves, garlic and green chillies
2. Heat oil. Add chopped vegetables. Fry for 2 to 3 minutes, then add the ground paste. Fry again for 2 to 3 minutes.
3. Add washed rice, sufficient water to cook rice and salt. Pressure cook till done.

VARIATION

Substitute chopped cabbage for coriander leaves.

AMLA RICE

Calories -500   *Serves -2*

Ingredients

Amla crushed – 25 gms   Asafoetida – a pinch
Rice – 100 gms   Curry leaves and coriander
Oil – 1 tbsp   leaves – a few
Mustard – 1 tsp   Salt – to taste
Red chillies – 2   Grated coconut – 1 tbsp (optional)

METHOD

1. Cook rice and season with oil, curry leaves, mustard, chillies and salt.
2. Add crushed amla and mix well.
3. Garnish with coriander leaves and grated coconut.

VARIATION

Grated raw mango can be used in place of amla during season.

PALAK RICE

Calories -508   *Serves -3*

Ingredients

Rice – 100 gms   Lime juice – 1 tbsp
Palak – 100 gms   Oil – 1 tbsp
                                  Salt – to taste

METHOD
1. Wash, chop and grind palak
2. Heat oil in a pan. Fry rice for 2 minutes.
3. Add water, salt and ground spinach. Cook till the rice is done.
4. Sprinkle lemon juice and mix well. Serve hot.

VARIATION
Chopped methi leaves can be used in place of palak.

SPROUTS KHICHADI

Calories -350   *Serves -4*

Ingredients

Sprouted moong – 50 gms   Pepper seeds – 15
Sprouted peas – 50 gms   Jeera – 1 tsp
Rice – 300 gms   Coconut – 1 tsp
Garlic – 6 clove   Salt – to taste
Chillies – 3

METHOD
Make a paste of garlic and chillies. Mix it with rice, sprouts and salt and pressure cook it. Season and garnish with coconut and coriander leaves.

AVALAKKI BISIBELE BATH

Calories -610   *Serves -3*

Ingredients

Rice flakes/Beaten rice – 100 gms

Green gram dal – 50 gms

Dry copra – 5 gms

Red chilli powder – ½ tsp

Daniya powder – 1 tsp

Garam masala – ½ tsp

Tomato – 50 gms

Salt – to taste

Oil – 5 gms

Mustard – ½ tsp

Curry leaves – a few

Water – 400 ml

METHOD

1. Roast green gram dal slightly and cook till it is soft.
2. Heat oil, add mustard, curry leaves, masala powder, cooked dal, tomato and salt.
3. Add water, cook till tomato is done. Add washed beaten rice. Cook till the flakes become soft.
4. Garnish with copra. Serve with raita.

VARIATION

Vegetables like carrot, beans and peas can be added.

VEGETABLE DALIA

Calories -520   *Serves -3*

Ingredients

Broken wheat – 100 gms   Salt – to taste
Beans – 25 gms   Coriander leaves – a few
Peas – 25 gms   Oil – 1 tbsp
Carrot – 25 gms   Mustard – 1 tsp
Curry leaves – a few

METHOD

1. Heat oil. Add mustard and curry leaves.
2. Roast broken wheat. Add to the seasoning. Add chopped vegetables.
3. Cook in pressure cooker, adding water and salt.
4. Garnish with coriander leaves.

Note: The consistency can be changed by adding water or milk.

WHEAT IDLI

Calories -935   *Serves -4*

Ingredients

Broken wheat – 200 gms   Salt – to taste
Carrot (grated) – 25 gms   Ginger crushed – a few
Coconut (grated) – 25 gms   Coriander leaves – a few
Curd – 200 ml

METHOD

1. Roast broken wheat. Add salt, water and curd till a paste like consistency is obtained. Keep aside for 30 minutes.
2. Add ginger, coriander leaves, carrot and coconut. Mix well.
3. Spread a ladle full on idli trays and steam for 15 minutes.
4. Serve hot with coconut chutney.

SABUDANA

SABUDANA KHICHADI

Calories -895   *Serves -5*

Ingredients

Sabudana – 200 gms
Ginger – 20 gms
Onion – 25 gms
Oil – 15 gms

Turmeric, mustard seeds
Curry and coriander leaves – a few
Salt – to taste

METHOD

1. Soak sago for about 1½ hours.
2. Chop onion, ginger and coriander leaves. Heat oil and add mustard, onion, curry leaves, ginger and turmeric.
3. Add soaked sago and salt. Cook till done by sprinkling water.
4. Serve with chutney or curds.

BARLEY

VEGETABLE BARLEY

Calories -730   *Serves -6*

Ingredients

Barley –200 gms
Carrot – 50 gms
Beans – 60 gms

Cabbage – 50 gms
Pepper, lemon juice and salt – to taste
Coriander leaves – a few

METHOD

1. Chop the vegetables and boil barley.
2. Half cook vegetables and add cooked barley and salt. Continue boiling for 5 to 10 minutes, adding required amount of water till done.
3. Add lime juice, pepper and coriander leaves. Serve hot.

WHEAT CHAPATI

Calories -341   *Serves -2*

Ingredients
Wheat flour – 100 gms
Salt – to taste

METHOD
1. Add salt to the wheat flour and make dough with water.
2. Divide into equal size balls and roll chapaties.
3. Bake it on a tava without adding oil.

WHEAT BESAN CHAPATI

Calories -715   *Serves -4*

Ingredients
Wheat flour – 100 gms
Besan flour – 100 gms
Salt – to taste

METHOD
Same as wheat chapati.

BARLEY CHAPATI

Calories -677   *Serves -4*

Ingredients
Wheat flour – 100 gms
Barley powder – 100 gms
Salt – to taste

METHOD
Same as wheat chapati.

SOYA CHAPATI

Calories -557   *Serves -3*

Ingredients

Wheat flour – 100 gms
Soya flour – 50 gms
Salt – to taste

METHOD
Same as wheat chapati.

DAL CHAPATI

Calories -400   *Serves -5*

Ingredients

Urad dal – 50 gms
Soya bean flour – 50 gms
Salt – to taste

METHOD
Boil urad dal and grind it to a paste. Mix it with besan flour and salt and make a soft dough. Roll and cook it.

Baked Delight

SOYA NIPPATTU

Calories -542   *Serves -2*

Ingredients

Soya flour – 40 gms
Wheat flour – 50 gms
Crushed peanuts – 25 gms
Ginger juice – 1 tsp
Sesame/Jeera – 1 tsp
Onion (chopped) – 25 gms
Yeast – 5 gms
Oil – 1 tsp
Salt – to taste

METHOD

1. Dissolve yeast in hot water and mix with flour.
2. Mix well all the above ingredients, divide into equal rounded portions, flatten each on greased baking tray.
3. Bake at 250° C for 15 minutes.

MASALA PURI

Calories -386   **Serves -2**

Ingredients

Wheat flour – 100 gms   Oil – 1 tsp
Jeera – ½ tsp   Salt – to taste
Pepper powder – ½ tsp   Coarsely powdered ⎤
Turmeric powder – ¼ tsp   coriander leaves, ⎬ 5 gms
                                          onion and yeast ⎦

METHOD
Same as Soya Nippattu.

YOGHURT SCONES

Calories -1020   **Serves -6**

Ingredients

Wheat flour – 200 gms   Curd – 200 gms
Salt – to taste   Oil – 15 gms
Baking powder – ½ tsp   Sesame seeds – 1 tsp (sprinkle)
Jaggery – 15 gms   Milk for brushing

METHOD
Same as Soya Nippattu.

GINGER BREAD

Calories -410   *Serves -2*

Ingredients

Wheat flour – 100 gms   *Green chilli – 1*
Mint – a few   *Yeast – ½ tsp*
Onion – 25 gms   *Ginger – 2 tsp (chopped)*
Salt – to taste   *Oil – 5 gms*

METHOD

Same as other baked products.

Note: Allow the dough to rise for 2-3 hours and put in bread moulds, and again leave for 1 hour, to rise.

BESAN BREAD

Calories -435   *Serves -3*

Ingredients

Whole wheat flour – 100 gms   *Salt – to taste*
Besan flour – 25 gms   *Ajwain – 1 tsp*
Yeast – ½ tsp

METHOD

Same as other baked products. Follow the procedure of ginger bread.

BAKED PURI

Calories -386   *Serves -2*

Ingredients

Wheat flour – 100 gms   Salt – to taste
Oil – 1 tsp   Ajwain – 1 tsp.

METHOD
Same as masala puri.

DILKUSH BAKED

Calories -420   *Serves -2*

Ingredients

Wheat flour – 100 gms   **For Stuffing**
Yeast – a pinch   Boiled vegetables –
Salt – to taste   cabbage, peas, beans and carrot
Oil – 1 tsp   – 50 gms
                                        Pepper powder and salt – to taste

METHOD
1. Make chapati dough with wheat flour and yeast.
2. Mix boiled vegetables with salt and pepper.
3. Divide the dough into equal size balls and flatten it.
4. Fill a portion of vegetable mixture and roll out the chappati.
5. Bake at 200°C for 15 minutes.
6. Serve with chutney or jam.

BAKED POOHA

Calories -840   **Serves -4**

Ingredients

Pooha – 100 gms
Chopped coriander – 1 tbsp
Green chilli – 1
Curd – 2 tbsp
Semolina – 3 tbsp

Jaggery – 1 tbsp
Salt – to taste
For seasoning:
Oil – 2 tsp
Mustard – ½ tsp
Asafoetida – a pinch

METHOD

Wash pooha in running water. Mix pooha, semolina, curds, jaggery, salt, coriander and green chilli.

Season it and leave for an hour to ferment.

Bake it at 200° C for 15 minutes.

CABBAGE TIKKI

Calories -448   **Serves -4**

Ingredients

Whole wheat flour – 100 gms
Yeast – ½ tsp
Cabbage – 50 gms

Salt – to taste
Jaggery – ½ tsp
Coriander leaves – a few

METHOD

1. Dissolve yeast in warm water and make a dough mixing all the ingredients (cabbage and coriander leaves chopped).
2. Mix well. Allow it to rest for 2 hours. Then divide into balls, flatten on the baking tray and bake at 215°C for 15 to 20 minutes.

RICE AND MOONG IDLI

Calories -435   *Serves -2*

Ingredients

Rice rava – 100 gms
Moong dal – 25 gms
Salt – to taste

METHOD

1. Soak moong dal for 5 to 6 hours and grind to a paste. Add salt.
2. Wash rice rava and add to ground moong dal paste. Allow it to ferment overnight.
3. Prepare idli as usual by steaming in idli moulds.

PALAK PURI

Calories -728   *Serves -7*

Ingredients

Wheat flour – 200 gms   *Grated coconut – 1 tsp*
Palak – 50 gms   *Yeast – a pinch*
Methi leaves – 25 gms   *Salt – to taste*

METHOD

Same as for Masala Puri.

MAIZE/CORN TIKKI

Calories -1224   *Serves -12*

Ingredients

Wheat flour – 300 gms   *Salt – to taste*
Corn (fresh) – 150 gms   *Pepper – ½ tbsp*
Carrot (grated) – 2 tbsp   *Yeast – a pinch*

METHOD
Same as for Masala Puri.

SOYABEAN TIKKI

Calories -812   *Serves -7*

Ingredients

Soyabean flour – 65 gms   *Jaggery – 1 tbsp*
Besan flour – 65 gms   *Chopped onion – 1 tbsp*
Wheat flour – 65 gms   *Yeast – a pinch*
Green chilli – 3

METHOD
Same as for Masala Puri.

Steamed Delight

BESAN DHOKLA

Calories -2977 *Serves -10*

Ingredients

Rice – 500 gms Coriander leaves – 1 bunch
Channa dal – 125 gms Mustard – 1 tsp
Urad dal – 100 gms Turmeric – a pinch
Oil – 15 gms Curds – 500 gms
Ginger – a little Salt – to taste

METHOD

1. Soak rice and dals separately for 5-6 hours. Then grind into a paste.
2. Mix curds and set aside for 5-6 hours.
3. Heat oil, add mustard and turmeric. Mix all the ingredients together and pour the mixture onto a greased tray. Steam it like idli for 15-20 minutes.
4. Cut into desired shape. Serve with chutney.

DAL VEGETABLES PANCAKE

Calories -3000   *Serves -10*

Ingredients
Rice suji (broken rice) – ½ kg
Black gram dal – ¼ kg
Beans – 100 gms

METHOD

1. Soak black gram dal for 8 hours and grind. Mix rice suji. Allow it to ferment overnight.
2. Mix salt, grated coconut, chopped green chillies and coriander leaves.
3. Make it into an idli batter, pour on idli moulds and steam.
4. Serve hot with chutney/sambar.

Steamed Vegetables

Steamed vegetables for patients

From the vast majority of vegetables of the flora kingdom, almost any number of permutation and combinations could be made and dishes prepared. Some of the commonly prepared and recommended vegetable combinations for the patients at the Institute of Naturopathy are given below. A unique feature of these preparations is the use of a very little amount of oil (sunflower oil/gingelly oil) for seasoning and a complete absence of spices - the latter have been incriminated as gastro-intestinal irritants. Any other combinations of vegetables could be made by adopting the same cooking methods.

While cooking, the following vital points must be adhered to:
1. Wash vegetables well before cutting.
2. Steam the vegetables in a cooker to minimise the loss of nutrients.
3. Avoid over-cooking and re-heating.
4. Never discard the cooked water. Hence use limited quantity of water.
5. Use tomatoes, coriander leaves in raw form.
6. Use jaggery or dates for sweetening.
7. After vegetables are cooked, add salt and pepper.
8. If desired, seasoning with oil, mustard and garlic could be done for improving the taste (optional).

Combinations:

1. Giya + palak + cumin seeds + oil + salt + turmeric.
2. French beans + carrot + tomatoes + mustard seeds + oil + salt + coriander leaves.
3. Cabbage + bengalgram dal + carrot + oil + mustard seeds + salt.
4. Cauliflower + methi leaves + tomatoes + oil + mustard seeds + turmeric + salt.
5. Snake gourd + ridge gourd + tomatoes + oil + mustard seeds + turmeric + salt.
6. Beetroot + soya + carrot + salt + pepper + coriander leaves.
7. Soyabean + knol - khol + carrot.
8. Rajmah + beans + tori + salt + pepper.
9. Peas + carrot + beetroot + salt + pepper.
10. Peas + khol khol + beans + salt + pepper.
11. Rajmah + carrot + knol-khol + salt + pepper.
12. Soyabean + kundri + beans + salt + pepper.
13. Kabuli channa + tori + carrot + salt + pepper.
14. Kabuli channa + cauliflower + beans + salt + pepper.
15. Kabuli channa + beetroot + kundri + salt + pepper.

Note: 100 gms of steamed vegetables provide 40-50 calories.

Ratio: 10 gms pulse + 90 gms mixed vegetables.

AMLA VEGETABLE MIX

Calories -107   **Serves -4**

Ingredients

Amla – 100 gms   Curds – 3 tbsp
Carrot – 100 gms   Salt – To taste
Cabbage –50 gms   Oil – 2 tbsp
Beetroot – 25 gms   Seasoning ingredients – a little
Coriander leaves – a few   Turmeric – 1/2 tsp

METHOD
1. Cut amla, sweet potato and carrot into cubes.
2. Shred cabbage and grate beetroot.
3. Mix amla, sweet potatoes, carrots and cabbage with salt.
4. Steam for 15-20 minutes in a bowl.
5. Season curds with oil, mustard, curry leaves and pour on the steamed vegetables.
6. Garnish with grated beetroot.

BANANA STEM CURRY

Calories -214   **Serves -7**

Ingredients

Banana stem – 1/2 kg (White   Salt – to taste
        portion)   Seasoning ingredients – a little
Coconut – 2 (250 gms)   mustard and a few curry leaves
Onion – 2 (75 gms)   Turmeric – a pinch
Oil – 15 gms

METHOD
1. Cut banana stem into pieces and immerse them in salt water for two hours. Then remove the sticky portion.

2. Heat oil, add seasoning ingredients. Add the remaining ingredients and a little water. Cook till banana stem becomes soft.
3. Remove from fire, serve with chapaties.

VARIATION
a. If desired, lemon juice may be added.
b. Amla (green variety) can be used along with banana stem.

BANANA FLOWER CURRY

Calories -1169   *Serves -4*

Ingredients

Banana flower – 1 bunch	*Salt – to taste*
Oil – 3 tbsp	*Seasoning ingredients – a little*
Onion – 100 gms	*mustard, turmeric and a few*
Coconut – 150 gms	*curry leaves*

METHOD
1. Cut the tender petals and immerse them in salt water. Wash three to four times.
2. Heat oil. Add all the ingredients. Cook for 20 minutes.

Sweets

SWEET DALIA (PORRIDGE)

Calories -600   *Serves -5*

Ingredients

Broken wheat – 100 gms
Cardamom powder – a pinch
Milk – 100 ml
Jaggery – 50 gm

METHOD

1. Boil broken wheat with milk and a little water till soft.
2. Add jaggery and cardamom powder, and boil for 5 minutes.
   Ideal as a breakfast item. Tasty to eat and healthy too.

VARIATIONS

Wheat can be roasted and then cooked. Jaggery can be replaced
by date pieces.

WHEAT HALWA

Calories -925   **Serves -8**

Ingredients

Wheat flour – 200 gms   Cardamom powder – a pinch
Jaggery – 25 gms   Ghee – 5 ml
Milk – 150 ml

METHOD

1. Roast wheat flour with ghee.
2. Add milk slowly to avoid lump formation. Then add jaggery and cardamom powder. Cook till the mixture leaves the sides of the pan.
3. Pour into a greased plate. When cool cut into desired shape.
4. Garnish with raisins and cashewnuts if desired.

WHEAT GERM LADDU

Calories -910   **Serves -8**

Ingredients

Wheat flour – 110 gms   Milk – to blend
Jaggery – 50 gms   Bengalgram flour – 100 gms

METHOD

1. Roast the two flours separately and add powdered jaggery. Mix well.
2. Add required amount of milk to make laddus.

RAGI HALWA

Calories -2826   *Serves -10*

Ingredients

Ragi – 500 gms   Ghee – 25 gms
Jaggery – 250 gms   Cardamom powder – 1 tsp

METHOD

1. Soak ragi in water for 6 hours. Grind it well by adding a little water.
2. Squeeze and extract the juice.
3. Boil the juice and add the grated jaggery. Stir constantly.

SABUDANA KHEER

Calories -1123   *Serves -8*

Ingredients

Sabudana – 200 gms   Milk – 200 ml
Jaggery – 75 gms   Cardamom – a pinch

METHOD

1. Soak sabudana in water for 1-1/2 hour. Boil it in water until well cooked.
2. Add the remaining ingredients and cook.
3. Easy to digest and relish - ideal for gastro-intestinal disorders like dysentry, diarrhoea and anorexia.

MOONG DAL KHEER

Calories -932   *Serves -5*

Ingredients

Moong dal – 100 gms   *Milk – 300 ml*
Jaggery – 100 gms   *Cardamoms, raisins, nuts – a few*

METHOD
1. Roast moong dal slightly and pressure cook.
2. Add milk and jaggery and boil till kheer consistensy is obtained.
3. Garnish with cardamom powder, nuts and raisins. Serve hot or cold.

SOYA PUMPKIN PUDDING

Calories -1065   *Serves -10*

Ingredients

Honey – 6 tbsp (100 gms)   *Pumpkin – 400 gms*
Whole wheat flour – 120 gms   *Pineapple juice - 15 ml (25 gms)*
Soya milk – 200 ml (50 gms)   *Cardamom powder – 1/4 tsp*

METHOD
1. Cook and mash the pumpkin. Blend all the ingredients. Bake in moderate oven at 180 C for 45 minutes.

CARROT HALWA

Calories -210   *Serves -1*

Ingredients

Carrot – 50 gms	*Ghee – 5 gms*
Milk – 100 ml	*Cardamom powder – a pinch*
Jaggery – 20 gms	*A few nuts and raisins for garnishing*

METHOD

1. Wash and grate carrots. Add milk and steam till cooked.
2. Add powdered jaggery and ghee. Cook on a low fire, stirring constantly till the mixture leaves the sides of the pan.
3. Pour on a greased plate, sprinkle cardamom powder and garnish with nuts and raisins. Cut into desired shape when cool.

SWEET POTATO HALWA

Calories -324   *Serves -2*

Ingredients

Sweet potato – 100 gms	*Ghee – 5 gms*
Jaggery – 30 gms	*Cardamom powder – a pinch*

METHOD

1. Wash and boil the potato with skin. Peel the skin and mash well. Add powdered jaggery and cook till the mixture becomes thick.
2. Add ghee and cardamom powder. Serve hot or cold.

TIL LADDU

Calories -396   *Serves -2*

Ingredients

Til – 50 gms
Jaggery – 30 gms
Cardamom – a pinch

METHOD

1. Roast til and cool. Pound it and add jaggery. Continue pounding till the mixture forms into a ball consistency.
2. Add cardamom powder and make into balls.

POACHED APPLE SLICES

Calories -130   *Serves -5*

Ingredients

Apple – 400 gms   *Orange – 1 (50 gm)*
Lemon – 1   *Water – 2 cups*
Jaggery – 100 gms

METHOD

1. Peel and core apples. Cut each apple into eight crescents.
2. Add jaggery into boiling water and when it is completely dissolved, add sliced apples into the syrup.
3. Cook till a fork pierces them.
4. Add orange and lemon juice and serve cold.

BANANA CAKE

Calories -400   *Serves -5*

Ingredients

Banana – 10	*Milk – 2 glasses (500 ml)*
Jaggery – 3/4 kg	*Cardamom powder – a pinch*
Wheat flour – 50 gms	*Raisins and cashewnuts – a few*
Ghee – 25 gms	

METHOD
1. Roast broken wheat.
2. Make jaggery syrup and strain.
3. Cut bananas into small pieces. Add cold milk, roasted broken wheat and jaggery syrup to banana pieces and cook the mixture thoroughly.
4. Add one-and-half tablespoon of ghee and continue cooking till the mixture thickens.
5. Transfer the mixture onto the greased plate, when cool, cut into desired shape and serve.

   Being easily digestible, it may be given even to the patients suffering from digestive problems.

DATES

A "DATE" WITH BANANA

Calories -263   *Serves -2*

Ingredients

Ripe banana – 2
Dates – 4 (20 gms)
Milk – 1 glass

METHOD:
1. Cut banana and dates into pieces and add water to blend.
2. Add milk and serve.

GUAVA CHEESE

Calories -1600   *Serves -20*

Ingredients

Guavas – 20 (1 kg) (fully   *Jaggery – 1/4 kg*
        ripened)   *Cardamom – a few pods*
Ghee – 1 tbsp

METHOD

1. Boil guavas till seed and pulp separate. Strain and take the pulp.
2. Make jaggery syrup of one thread consistency.
3. Add the cooked pulp. Stir constantly till the paste thickens.
4. Spread onto a greased plate, cut into desired shape. Serve cold.

GUAVA SWEET AND SOUR

Calories -510   *Serves -5*

Ingredients

Guavas – 500 gms   *Salt – to taste*
Tomato – 1/2 kg   *Turmeric – a pinch*
Oil – 2 tsp   *Coconut – 1 tbsp*
Mustard – 1/2 tsp   *Coriander leaves – a few*

METHOD

1. Cut guavas and tomatoes into uniform cubes.
2. Heat oil, add mustard, guavas, tomatoes, salt and turmeric.
3. Stir occasionally till it is cooked.
4. Pour it into a vessel. Garnish with coriander leaves and coconut gratings.

HONEY

SHAHI HONEY

Calories -129   *Serves -4*

Ingredients

Ashgourd – 500 gms
Honey – 25 gms
Lime – 1

METHOD

1. Cut ashgourd into small pieces. Prick these pieces with a fork and boil in water to which lime juice has been added.
2. Cook till the inner core is softened. Then dry the pieces.
3. Soak the dried pieces in thick honey syrup for 6 hours. Serve cold.

CREAMY HONEY PUDDING

Calories -1084   *Serves -5*

Ingredients

Rice – 4 tbsps	*Cinnamon – 1/2 tsp*
Milk – 3/4 lt	*Salt – 1/2 tsp*
Honey – 1/2 cup (126 ml)	*Raisins – 1/2 cup*

METHOD

1. Wash rice. Add the remaining ingredients to the rice. Pour the mixture into a greased dish.
2. Bake for 2-3 hours on low temperature in the oven at 200 C.
3. Serve hot or cold.

153

SWEET DALIA (POPULAR AS PORRIDGE)

Calories -604   *Serves -6*

Ingredients

Broken wheat – 100 gms   Milk – 100 gms
Jaggery – 50 gms   Cardamom powder – a pinch

METHOD

1. Cook the broken wheat. When cooked, add jaggery and milk.
2. Add cardamom powder and mix well.
   Ideal for breakfast. Tasty to eat and little effort is involved to introduce in daily diet by the families.

VARIATION

Instead of adding jaggery, dalia may be cooked along with date pieces.

RAGI MALT/RAGI PORRIDGE

Calories -540   *Serves -5*

Ingredients

Ragi – 100 gms
Honey – 3 tsp
Milk – 250 ml

METHOD

1. Germinate the ragi grains till the shoot is about 1 km long. Roast and powder ragi sprouts.
2. Add milk and stir. Honey or jaggery may be used for sweetening.
   It is nourishing and refreshing drink especially for growing children and convalescents.

BANANA SWEET AND SOUR

Calories -140   *Serves -5*

Ingredients

Bananas – 10 (half ripe)	*Coriander leaves – 1 bunch*
Oil – 2 tsp	*Mustard – 1/2 tbsp*
Tomato – 500 gms	*Turmeric – a pinch*
Coconut – 5 gms (fresh)	

METHOD

1. Cut bananas and tomatoes into cubes.
2. Heat oil. Add mustard seeds, bananas and tomatoes. Add salt and turmeric.
3. Cook, stirring occasionally for 10 minutes.
4. Remove from fire, garnish with coriander leaves and coconut gratings.

VARIATION

a. Tamarind can be substituted for tomatoes.
b. Guavas can be substituted for bananas.

Beverages

Drinks and Appetisers

The natural goodness of fruits and vegetables is best extracted as juices.

Besides being alkaline in nature and a mine of water soluble vitamins and minerals, juices have an additional advantage of being consumed in amounts much more than is possible to consume the fruits or vegetables as such.

An indefinite number of delightful and imaginative combination could be obtained from this indispensable food group.

COOL CUCUMBER

Calories -230   *Serves -2*

Ingredients
Tomato – 100 gms
Cucumber – 1 kg
Sesame powder – 1 tbsp
Salt – to taste

METHOD
1. Blend tomato and cucumber, setting aside some cucumber pieces for garnishing. Add powdered sesame and salt to taste.
2. Before serving garnish with cucumber pieces.

AAM RAS (MANGO JUICE)

Calories -260   *Serves -2*

Ingredients

Ripe mango – 250 gms   Jaggery – 20 gms
Water – 500 ml   Cardamom – a pinch
                              Salt – a pinch

METHOD

1. Boil mango till soft. Remove the pulp.
2. Dissolve jaggery in water and strain to pulp. Liquidise in a mixie. Add cardamom powder and salt. Serve cold.

PAPAYA SHAKE

Calories -169   *Serves -1*

Ingredients

Ripe papaya – 200 gms   Ripe banana – 50 gms
Honey – 1 tbsp   Cardamom powder – a pinch

METHOD

1. Blend the pulp of papaya and banana by adding a little water. Add honey and cardamom powder. Serve cold. It is a rich "golden" yellow drink, both appetising and nourishing.

SWEET ELIXIR

Calories -250   *Serves -1*

Ingredients

Carrot juice – 30 ml
Honey – 10 ml
Sunflower seeds – a pinch

METHOD

Powder sunflower seeds. Mix with carrot juice and honey. Serve cool.

FRUIT COCKTAILS

Calories -765   *Serves -5*

Ingredients

Grapes – 400 gms   *Orange – 250 gms*
Pineapple – 500 gms   *Honey – 30 ml*
Apple – 150 gms   *Salt and pepper – to taste*

METHOD

1. Chop apples and pineapples. Squeeze the juice of orange.
2. Extract the juice of pineapple and apple by adding one cup of water, and strain. Blend grapes and strain separately.
3. Mix all the juices. Just before serving add honey, salt and pepper.

SWEET FRUIT DELIGHT

Calories -832   *Serves -5*

Ingredients

Fresh apple juice – 250 ml   *Coconut milk – 125 ml*
Apple pieces – 100 gms   *Green grapes – 100 gms*

METHOD
1. Blend apple juice and coconut milk. Serve with apple slices and grapes floating on top.

ORANGE CARROT SHERBET

Calories -92   *Serves -2*

Ingredients

Carrot juice – 50 ml   *Lime juice – 5 ml*
Orange juice – 50 ml   *Jaggery – 10 gms*
Tomato juice – 25 ml   *Mint leaves – a few*

METHOD
Mix all the ingredients, strain and serve with a few mint leaves on top.

WHEAT DRINK

Calories -320   *Serves -2*

Ingredients

Wheat germ – 50 gms   *Jaggery – 10 gms*
Milk – 200 gms   *Water – 200 ml*

METHOD
1. Boil milk and water, add wheat germ. Cook till it becomes soft. Add jaggery, continue cooking for 5 minutes. Serve hot.

VARIATION
Grind wheat germ, adding water. Add jaggery, boil or drink cold.

159

SOYA MILK

Calories -160   *Serves -1*

Ingredients

Soya – 20 gms
Jaggery – 20 gms
Water – 200 ml

METHOD

Soak soya overnight. Remove the skin and grind it in the morning to a paste. Dilute with water and boil. Add jaggery or honey and serve hot.

RELAXING PUNCH

Calories -140   *Serves -2*

Ingredients

Honey – 20 ml   *Lemon juice – 100 ml*
Orange juice – 100 ml   *Apple – 100 gms*

METHOD

Blend all the ingredients in the mixer and cool in the fridge. Serve with or without ginger juice.

CLEANSING DRINK

Calories -Negligible

Ingredients

Saunf – 1 tsp   *Mint leaves – 8 to 10*
Ajwain – 1/2 tsp   *Rock salt – a pinch*
                                   Water – 300 ml

METHOD

1. Boil saunf, ajwain and mint leaves in 2½ cup water. Boil well to get 1¼ cup water.
2. Strain, add rock salt. Serve hot with a piece of lemon.

Calorie Content

The calorie is a measurement of energy content in food. We need energy from food to live and carry out our daily activities and when we eat more than the energy required, the excess is stored in the body as fat. So we become overweight.

To stay slim and healthy, we should balance the energy input with the energy output. This chart may be used to check the approximate calorie content of food we eat every day.

Sl. No.	Recipe	Portion/Size	Calorie Value
I.	**Cereals/Rice/Bread/Noodles**		
	Plain rice (cooked)	100 gms	175
	Curd rice	100 gms	250
	Chapati (one piece)	20 gm	70
	Paratha (plain)	one	150
	Paratha (stuffed)/Masala dosa	one	200
	Dosa (plain)	one	150
	Puri	one	95
	Bread (plain)	2 slices	154
	Brown bread (1 piece)	20 gm	40
	Samosa/Toast with Butter/Idli (45 gm)	medium	100
	Vada Sambar	2 nos.	140
	Baked masala puri (1)	75 gm	188
	Baked noodles	100 gm	175
	Dokla (steamed) (1 piece)	35 gm	80
	Soya nippattu (1)	60 gm	233

	Soyabean tikki (1 no.)	45 gm	127
	Fresh maize tikki (1 no.)	45 gm	109
	Cabbage tikki (1 no.)	85 gm	106
	Palak puri (1 no.)	45 gm	112
	Yoghurt scones (1 no.)	85 gm	141
II.	SALADS	100 gms	20-25
III.	FRUITS		(100 gms edible portion)
	Apple		59
	Apricot		53
	Beal fruit		137
	Banana (ripe)		116
	Cherries		64
	Dates (dried)		317
	Grapes (Black)		58
	Grapes (Green)		71
	Grapefruit/Musk melon		17
	Guava		51
	Sweet lime		35
	Mango ripe/ Wood apple		34
	Water melon		16
	Raisins	100 gms	308
	Orange		48
	Papaya (raw)		32
	Peach		50
	Pear/plum		52
	Pineapple		46
	Pomegranate		65
	Sapota		98
	Custard apple		104
IV.	JUICES		
	Lemon juice (half a lemon)	10 gms	6
	Lemon juice with honey	250 ml	22
	Honey water	one spn. (10 gm)	32
	Tender coconut water		52
	Carrot juice		120
	Mausambi juice		160
	Papaya juice		50
	Grape juice		115
	Orange juice		145

	Pineapple juice		
	Sugarcane juice		
	Fruit Cocktail canned	120 gms	100
	Tomato juice		60
	Custard apple juice		70
V.	**BAKED/BOILED VEGETABLES**	100 gms	50-80
VI.	**SOUPS**	250 ml	16-35
VII.	**CHUTNEY**		
	Chutney mint	tbsp	15-20
	Hara dhania	tbsp	5-10
VIII.	**RAITHAS**	100 gms	50-80
IX.	**SPROUTS**	50 gms	
	Groundnut		178
	Bengal gram		100
	Green gram		112
	Wheat/Bajra		85
X.	**VEGETABLES**	(100 gms edible portion)	
(a)	**Leafy Vegetables**		
	Agathi		93
	Bathua		30
	Cabbage		27
	Celery		37
	Coriander leaves		44
	Curry leaves		108
	Methi leaves		49
	Lettuce		21
	Mint		48
	Parsley		87
	Radish leaves		28
	Spinach		26
	Carrot greens		77
	Beet greens		46
	Onion Stalk		41
(b)	**Roots and Tubers**		
	Beet root		43
	Carrot		48
	Colocasia/Potato		97
	Onion (Big)		50
	Radish		17
	Sweet potato		120
	Tapioca		157

Turnip		29
Yam		111

(c) Other Vegetables

Ashgourd/Pumpkin		10
Bitter gourd/Pumpkin		25
Tinda		21
Tomato green		23
French beans		26
Brinjal/Capsicum		24
Cauliflower		30
Cucumber		13
Lady's finger		35
Papaya green		27

XI. MILK & MILK PRODUCTS

Milk (buffalo)	One cup	210
Milk (Cow)	One cup	130
Cow milk with honey (tbsp)	One cup	162
Milk shake	250 ml	210
Ghee	one tbsp	50
Butter	one tbsp	35
Butter milk	250 ml	40
Soya milk	250 ml	260

XII. SUGAR/SWEETS/SPREADS

Sugar	one tbsp	20
Honey	two tbsp	31
Milk chocolate	two pcs (40 gms)	212
Ice cream (Vanila)	1 cup	160
Rassogulla	medium size 1	120

XIII. CAKES/PASTRIES/SNACKS

Fruit cake	(50 gms) 1 wedge	177
Choco cake	(55 gms) 1 wedge	251
Custard	(135 gms) one	374
Apple Pie	(85 gms) one	263
Popcorn	(250 gms) 1 pkt	148
Tea/Coffee with milk and sugar	one cup	50
Salt biscuits	4 nos.	100
Cream crackers	3 nos.	100
Potato crisp (35 gms)	1 pkt	187

XIV. COOKING OILS

Soya/Groundnut	3 tbsp	120
Sunflower/Safflower	3 tbsp	130

Protein Content of Different Foods

Recipe			Protein (gms)
CEREALS			
Rice (raw milled)	-	100 gms	6.8
Wheat	-	100 gms	11.8
Wheat flour (whole)	-	100 gms	12.1
Wheat bread (white)	-	100 gms	7.8
Wheat bread (brown)	-	100 gms	8.8
PULSE			
Bengalgram dal	-	100 gms	20.8
Bengalgram (roasted)	-	100 gms	22.5
Blackgram dal	-	100 gms	24.0
Cowpea	-	100 gms	24.0
Greengram dal	-	100 gms	24.5
Redgram dal	-	100 gms	22.30
Soyabean	-	100 gms	42.20
NUTS AND OIL SEEDS			
Almond	-	100 gms	20.80
Cashewnut	-	100 gms	21.20
Groundnut	-	100 gms	25.30
MILK AND MILK PRODUCTS			
Cow's milk	-	100 gms	3.2

Buffalo's milk	-	100 gms	4.3
Khoa	-	100 gms	22.3
Skimmed milk powder	-	100 gms	25.8

LEAFY VEGETABLES AND OTHER VEGETABLES

Agathi	-	100 gms	8.4
Amaranthus	-	100 gms	5.9
Colocasia leaves	-	100 gms	13.7
Drumstick leaves	-	100 gms	6.7
Beans	-	100 gms	7.4
Double beans	-	100 gms	8.3

FRUITS

Lime	-	100 gms	1.5
Passion fruit	-	100 gms	1.2
Banana	-	100 gms	1.2
Pomegranate	-	100 gms	1.6
Wood apple	-	100 gms	7.1
Raisins	-	100 gms	1.8

Courtesy : "Nutritive Value of Indian Foods"

Trifala for removing गल्द from stomach.

50 ml. — तिल तेल
pm 20 ghee
1 mm cinamon oil
1 ml - Ajwain oil.

nil grain oil.

166